STAY OUT OF THE HOSPITAL

by

Nathaniel Welsher Boyd III, D.O.

DORRANCE & COMPANY • *Philadelphia and Ardmore, Pa.*

Library of Congress Catalog Card Number: 76-39730

I wish to dedicate this book to that small group of osteopathic physicians and surgeons who year after year have used their political connections to get themselves appointed and reappointed to the Pennsylvania State Board of Osteopathic Medical Examiners, in the cases of three men, for twenty years or more. Their constant harassment and persecution have helped me to achieve the determination and energy to write this book. So at long last they have performed a useful function.

If a man does not keep pace with his companions, perhaps it is because he hears a different drummer. Let him step to the music which he hears, however measured or far away.

Thoreau, *Walden*

Who steals my purse steals trash . . .
But he that filches from me my good name
Robs me of that which not enriches him
And makes me poor indeed.

Shakespeare, *Othello*

I have little sympathy for those who assert that no further improvement is to be expected in surgical technic.

The surgeon must not zealously insist on continuing the treatment of conditions which experience will prove, from time to time, can be better managed by other than surgical means. Science, like time, marches on. Progress beyond our wildest imaginings is coming.

J. Tate Mason, Past President
of the American Medical
Association

Acknowledgments

I wish to thank Gary Moore, whose education at Johns Hopkins University equipped him well to help me with the language and organization of this book, and my patients, whose encouragement has bolstered me during the hard times an individual is bound to face when he works in a profession controlled by an Establishment opposed to his views.

Contents

Foreword

In my travels to college and university campuses around the United States, I have been astounded by the huge buildings erected to house libraries and lecture halls for the communication of knowledge, knowledge which is taught because it is useful, helpful to humanity. And yet there is knowledge—valuable knowledge—that is never taught and never learned in those halls, knowledge that is deliberately excluded.

For twenty-five years I have labored in a unique field outside the regular medical orthodoxy. I specialize in the ambulatory office treatment of almost all rectal disease, 85 percent of all hernias, and the majority of enlarged prostate glands, for which men customarily go to the hospital for surgery. My patients have been satisfied, and I know that my work is sound. I knew from the beginning, however, that because I had broken with orthodoxy, recognition and professional acceptance would never be mine. I knew that the knowledge I possessed and practiced would always be banned from the university lecture halls. As the years passed, many of my patients suggested that I write a book—this book. This publication will serve as the justification of my path, the record of my success, and the statement of what I have learned. I feel I have something to say in it that has never been said to the public before.

Pioneering is never an easy task, but the satisfaction of knowing that people gladly come hundreds of miles to avoid hospital surgery is rewarding far beyond dollars and cents. It has been most satisfying to successfully treat, in a few office visits, people who were deathly afraid of hospital surgery and who would live with a painful and debilitating condition for the rest of their lives rather than submit to the trauma of a hospital operation.

It is sad that we have become so much the prisoners of our health insurance that patients are submitting to hospital surgery they do not want because they feel they have to recoup their investment. No physicians want to learn to cure these patients without hospital surgery because the fees for office treatment are small or nonexistent, whereas the fees paid by insurance companies for hospital surgery are large. As a result, the system is very effectively going to consign to oblivion treatment methods that deserve a far better fate. The facts are recorded in this book.

I give my heartfelt thanks to the many patients and friends who have sustained me over the years of frustration while I tried to gain acceptance of my work by the medical establishment—opposed all the while by other doctors and the medical insurance companies. To those few physicians, most of them now dead, who taught me my art, not in lecture halls but in their offices, I owe a debt of gratitude I can never repay.

I still hope that this work will survive and spread and someday be taught in those huge buildings on university campuses—although I doubt that it will. I love the work and I love its challenges. The satisfaction I receive from it is great. I regret that it cannot receive the recognition and acceptance of other practitioners and surgeons. Their rejection of it is a loss not only to me but to them as well, and, most unfortunately, to the poor suffering public, which is denied the knowledge that such treatment even exists.

I

Is There a Doctor Shortage?

It is widely held in the United States that we have a doctor shortage. This is bunk.

Show me an overly busy doctor and I will show you, 90 percent of the time, a man who has magnified small complaints, helping to make his patients into hypochondriacs who spend too much of their salaries running to the doctor. At least three fourths of the patients in the average doctor's office are there for a routine checkup or for some very minor complaint.

Recently a medical journal told of a doctor from New York City who was bored with his practice and relocated in a small town in Maine. He was thrilled with the number of new patients he was seeing and with the interesting pathology he found in his new practice. "Before," he said, "so much of my time was spent seeing people for routine checkups." It makes one wonder whether many doctors are seeing people who do not really need to be seen at all. The incidence of manufactured and carefully cultivated practices in the United States is very high.

There is no shortage of doctors in this country, but there is certainly a poor distribution of doctors. Why is this so? The ratio of people to physicians in the United States is about 700 to 1, but it is as high as 4,000 to 1 in some areas, while in the suburbs of the big cities it is as low as 250 people to 1 physician. Of course, most doctors like the entertainment, fancy restaurants, and bright lights of the big city. And it is also true that cultural advantages and better

1

medical consultations are present in the large urban areas. This situation has been with us for a long while, and no solution has been found.

My first solution would be to give preferential medical school admission to those students who come from rural areas with real doctor shortages. Such students are much more likely to practice in these areas once they become physicians than city-born physicians.

Another method would be to make every doctor practice for five years where he is really needed. Those who want solutions but are unwilling to make sacrifices would of course balk at this suggestion. But such service would be a small price to pay for the privilege of being a member of a profession, highly respected for thousands of years, which gives enormous personal satisfaction to its practitioners. If this plan were put into effect, I think, many would be surprised to see these doctors decide that small communities are really good locations for living, raising families, and practicing medicine. Many would decide to stay where they enjoy life and where they are needed.

In the ghettos of the big cities there is also a shortage of doctors. Medicaid has partially cured this doctor shortage in the cities by reimbursing doctors at the rate of $5.70 per patient visit. This sounds like a small payment until one realizes the production-line type of care these doctors are giving the poor souls who come to them as patients. Not only do they see as many as 150 patients a day, but these physicians have also been known to falsify records, asserting they have seen a patient eighty or ninety times when in truth they have never laid eyes on the patient but have merely gotten the patient's name from a relative. The 150 people they do see in one day must receive quite shabby treatment. My considered opinion is that no conscientious physician can give reasonable care to more than forty people a day, in any type of practice. Nonetheless, government figures released in 1975 show that 215 doctors in the United States made over $100,000 from Medicaid in the preceding year. One New York doctor received $415,156 from Medicaid for a year of treating the poor and indigent.

An especially sad and ironic feature of the Medicaid situation is that many in America's forgotten lower middle class, with incomes of $7,000 to $15,000 a year, cannot afford to go to the doctor, although their tax money is being used to pay for the visits of poor people. The rich can afford it and the poor can get care for nothing, leaving approximately fifty percent of the people up the well-known creek. But considering the quality of care a patient gets when he is one of fifteen seen in an hour, perhaps those who don't go to the doctor are better off than those who do.

While I was taking a course in rectal disease treatment in Boston, I met a so-called physician from California who bragged to me that he recently had seen ninety-eight people in one day. Thank God he is in California; I want him far away from me. I suppose this statement was made to make me think that he was a great doctor. It had the opposite effect.

When I was a medical student some of my classmates kept talking about going to the ghetto to practice for a few years. I was naive enough to think they were great humanitarians, until three years later, when I saw them all far ahead of the rest of us financially and realized that they were profiteering from government medical funds. Their motivation was not altruism but greed. After a few years of cashing in on these government-subsidized medical plans in the ghetto they could move to the suburbs, where life was more pleasant. Though doctors were too plentiful in the suburbs, these men could cultivate a practice by selling the well-heeled and medically insured suburbanites medical treatments and surgery they did not need.

I am conjuring an image of physicians as greedy men. Unfortunately the desire to make money, lots of money, has all too great a part in the motivation of young men and women choosing medicine as a career. One unfortunate result of this emphasis on money is the rush to get into medical and surgical specialties while the practice of general medicine becomes extinct. Medical education encourages this trend, emphasizing the diagnosis and treatment of rare diseases and giving too little attention to common and minor complaints. Too much emphasis is put on using highly sophisticated equipment and expensive lab tests and not enough on history taking and reliance on the doctor's five—and yes, even six—senses. Another result of the physician's putting emphasis on his income is, of course, the willingness of doctors to perform unnecessary treatments and operations.

It is heartening to be able to report that I have known men who, I am sure, went into medicine to get rich, but, somewhere along the line, changed. A wonderful thing happened, and they began to show a compassion and concern I did not think they possessed. These men have turned out to be wonderful physicians who made one proud to be their colleague. But greed exists in the minds of most men, and some people continue to go into medicine because its financial rewards, as we all know, can be great.

We do not need more doctors more interested in their own profits than in good health care. We do not need more doctors who steer patients to physician-owned pharmacies where prices are elevated and often more than fifty percent of the exorbitant prescription price goes into the doctor's pocket. Of course, this is an extreme depth that most never sink to, and we must not lose track of the fact that over 50 percent of all doctors are straight as an arrow. But there is greed controlling much medical practice in the United States, and a surprising amount of ignorance, too. I do not believe that increasing the number of physicians will do any good for the health of the people or the wealth of the nation. More doctors would merely increase the competition in securing patients and performing operations. More doctors, both competent and incompetent, would continue to find ways of making a dishonest living at the expense of those they are sworn to help. The answer, of course, would be to get rid of the bad apples at the beginning.

Psychological testing to determine a potential physician's motivation has been tried but is very difficult and at best unreliable. And as in the case of those doctors who have changed for the better, a doctor's motivation changes as he goes through life. Such a test, even if accurate today, would not necessarily show the motivation of an individual twenty years from now.

Although we could use more doctors motivated by the interest of their patients and the challenge of their work, it is a change in quality and not in quantity that we require. In fact, it has to be recognized that in many forms of practice we already have too many physicians.

4

The surgical profession itself recognizes that there are far too many men in the United States doing surgery. A panel whose chairman was Harvard's Dr. Francis D. Moore found that for 94,000 United States doctors surgical operations form a major part of their professional activity. This figure represents over 30 percent of all active practitioners, more than twice the percentage of surgeons in most countries.

The same study declares that the number of surgical training positions offered in the United States—16,000—is excessive by any standard, and concludes that one-third of this number would be adequate. This expert opinion notwithstanding, a recent study published in *Medical Economics* (August 9, 1976) estimates that the number of general surgeons in the U.S. will be *nearly doubled* by 1980 and *nearly tripled* by 1990. Incidentally, the study which Dr. Moore oversaw also concluded that there was no scientific evidence to indicate that board-certified surgeons do better work than noncertified surgeons.

Dr. George Crile, Jr., emeritus consultant at the Cleveland Clinic, discussed unnecessary or "inappropriate" operations in the August 1 issue of *Modern Medicine.* Having isolated three distinct classes of inappropriate operations—those inappropriate for the disease, those inappropriate for the patient, and those performed by a surgeon inappropriately trained to do them—Dr. Crile suggested that hospitals stop appointing new fee-for-service surgeons and limit their new appointments to salaried surgeons who would be needed and would therefore be kept busy. Such a practice would have benefits beyond the high standard of surgery that could thus be attained. It would help to eliminate unnecessary operations hustled up by surgeons to keep their income flowing.

Government and academic surgeons tend to do remarkably fewer operations—88 to 104 a year—than fee-for-service surgeons, who do 171 to 223 major operations a year. Thus, surgeons on salary do only one-half as much surgery as surgeons who stand to gain by performing more surgery. Is this extra surgery unnecessary? Probably. No one has ever suggested that surgeons on salary are not doing enough surgery.

Not only is there far too much surgery being done—perhaps 50

5

percent more than necessary—but of the necessary surgery that is being done probably 30 percent could be done in facilities without all the expensive sophisticated equipment that large hospitals seem to accumulate whether they need it or not. Early in 1970 two Phoenix, Arizona, anesthesiologists, John L. Ford and Wallace A. Reed, opened an independent "surgicenter" and soon claimed a saving of $130 for each patient admitted. The most frequently performed operations were diagnostic dilatation and curettage of the uterus, muscle operations on the eye, and the removal of cataracts. Other work they found congenial to this facility included rectal surgery, tonsil surgery, and removal of almost all skin abnormalities. But this type of surgical treatment in a small independent facility was not the first of its kind: I have been doing such surgery on patients with all rectal diseases, hernias, and prostate disorders since 1951.

In May of 1975 *Medical Economics Magazine* reported that after five years only twenty of these surgicenters existed in the United States. This slow rate of growth can be attributed to several causes, all in the final analysis reducible to one fact and one fact only. Such facilities hurt the pocketbooks of doctors who have been able to keep them from growing and spreading. The difficulties they face are numerous.

1. Physicians worry that these centers or clinics will take over minor procedures usually done in their offices.

2. Critics claim that life-threatening emergencies can arise that these facilities may prove unable to handle. The Phoenix center, however, reports that in 26,500 procedures there has not been a single fatality or emergency transfer to a hospital.

3. More than four years went by before Medicare would honor the Phoenix center claims. To this day in the author's clinic Medicare pays less than one third of the cost of most claims submitted.

4. Blue Cross and Blue Shield officials voice fears that the spread of such clinics will aggravate hospital bed surpluses. Of course they will. But what happened to all the talk about a hospital bed *shortage?*

5. Critics—speaking candidly—claim that facilities such as the

6

Phoenix surgicenter and my clinic, in Loganville, Pennsylvania, will skim the cream off the surgical milk bottle. Anyone who accuses us of that is in effect admitting that the potential patients of our facilities either do not require hospital surgery or are now paying more than they should for hospital services.

A chief of surgery at a well-known children's hospital was recently asked why he did not do all his hernia repairs on children on an in-and-out basis. His reply was to ask if the questioner was out of his mind. Most of the surgery his department gets, he explained, is hernia repair. If they did all hernias on an in-and-out basis they would lose half of their service and the beds would be taken over by the medical department. This kind of self-interest in which hospital beds become symbols of status and power is one of the reasons medical politicians will fight any attempt to prevent hospitalization, even if they know that avoidance of hospitalization is a good thing for the physically suffering and economically hurting patient.

Another factor stunting the growth of in-and-out surgicenters is the insistence of insurance companies that the patient stay in the hospital overnight. Otherwise, they will not pay for his surgery. What their rationale for this policy is I do not know, unless it is to keep hospital beds filled. And since hospital rules demand a complete blood count, urinalysis, and chest X ray of every patient, the patient is subjected to generally unnecessary and always expensive lab work. Most patients are thus forced to spend two, three, or even four days in a hospital for an uncomplicated operation requiring less than one hour.

Besides the obvious savings in dollars, there are several advantages in going to a surgicenter such as that in Phoenix and my clinic in Loganville:

1. There is less, if any, waiting time when office surgery is needed than there is when a hospital bed and the collaboration of institutional specialists and technicians is required.

2. There is less trauma and anxiety for patients. Once patients know a procedure must be performed, they want to get it over with as soon as possible instead of worrying about it for a week or two or three. Patients often have apprehensions about having to stay in

a hospital, apprehensions which persist no matter how much the doctor tries to allay them. This apprehension is of course eliminated when hospitalization is not required.

3. There is less danger of cross-infection. Patients admitted to crowded wards often contact an upper respiratory infection or enteritis and take it home to their families. My patients are not exposed to infections that are often prevalent in hospital wards, and my patients, in turn, do not expose other hospital patients to infections they may be carrying.

4. There is no wasted preoperative and postoperative time away from home including elaborate tests and perhaps a needless stay over the weekend before surgery. During such stays most doctors feel compelled to visit each patient regularly whether there is good reason to or not, and they charge for these visits. Thus the patient often ends up paying three or more doctors a fee each day of his incarceration. Under the clinic system only one doctor needs to see the patient only a few minutes, while the actual treatment is being given.

Treatment in a clinic does not, as hospital treatment does, require the services of the internal medicine specialist, the pathologist, the radiologist, the intern who goes over charts and writes daily progress notes, and the resident who oversees the intern. It does not require the services of nurses, kitchen aides, and a housekeeping staff.

American medical and surgical patients are being overtreated by expensive specialists using elaborate equipment, performing unnecessary hospital surgery, and encouraging needless office visits. The remedy for this situation is a better educated public, a public that can think more for itself instead of being in such awe of the exclusive healing powers of doctors that it runs for professional treatment each time it cuts a finger, sprains an ankle, or catches a cold. Most upper respiratory ailments, as the saying goes, run seven days if treated by the patient and a week if treated by a doctor. The shot of penicillin, by the way, that many doctors administer for ten dollars in such cases, is acquired by the doctor for about six cents. Additionally, penicillin should never be given for a virus infection, which is of course the causative agent in the common cold. It does not cure the cold but only builds up the body's resistance to the antibiotic so that it will be less effective later if it is really needed for some bacteriological disease against which penicillin is the proper agent.

If there were a real doctor shortage, physicians wouldn't have time to give such expensive, not to mention inappropriate, treatment for ailments that could be handled by para-professionals or go just as well without treatment.

The proof of the pudding may be seen in the practice of the pseudospeciality known as "bariatrics." Bariatricians are doctors who take overweight people and submit them to a batch of tests, which they pay for and which seldom rule any of them out as patients. They are then likely to give these people thyroid extract and powerful drugs such as diuretics, digitalis, and amphetamines—all useful preparations if properly used but harmful when used recklessly. The diuretics rapidly take water out of the body, giving the patient a sudden first-week weight loss which encourages him or her to stick with the program. In such "programs," the patients part with three hundred to five hundred dollars but seldom maintain any weight loss for more than one or two years. They lose money and they lose bodily health by subjecting themselves to drugs that are in no way appropriate.

Unfortunately—and I hate to say this—the number of osteopathic physicians in this work is far higher than the four percent that they constitute of the national physician population. The founders of osteopathic medicine would turn over in their graves if they knew this, because, as you probably know, one of the original objections of osteopathy to conventional medical practice was that conventional doctors were overdrugging the public.

Do the state boards of examiners discipline these men in any way? Of course not. In most states there are thirty or forty men doing this work, and in numbers there is strength. The gutless boards would never dare attack a large group of physicians, but if one lonely individual develops treatment methods that deprive the other doctors of a little of their excessive incomes he had better look out.

A much more sensible way to take off weight would be to

develop new eating habits. Weight Watchers and TOPS (Take Off Pounds Sensibly) are excellent lay groups that offer less dangerous and more intelligent methods of obesity control.

The present medical practice of "bariatrics" can in most cases be judged both harmful and unnecessary. Their means are harmful, and the specialization of these greedy men in a field whose short-lived results are primarily cosmetic, is a woeful luxury in our society, inconsistent with the claim that we have a doctor shortage.

Some countries do need more doctors. That is why underdeveloped nations such as Iran, India, Pakistan, and the Philippines send young men and women to the United States for medical training. Here they take D.O. and M.D. degrees or pursue advanced training in rigorous specialties such as heart and great-vessel surgery. All too often, however, these people do not go home to practice medicine or surgery, but instead stay here for the rest of their lives. Why does our State Department allow this? Not only do these physicians fail to alleviate critical shortages in their own countries, but they also increase the competition among doctors for patients in this country, competition which results in doctor visits and surgical procedures performed not because they are necessary for patient well-being but because they are necessary to keep doctors busy.

The medical professional is cynical on the point of how many doctors the public will support. In the last decade the number of students in U.S. medical schools has doubled, from 26,000 in 1965 to 53,000 in 1974. In a recent issue of *Modern Medicine* (January 1976) these figures were used in connection with the question of whether we are producing too many doctors. No, said one physician, the capacity of the public to absorb additional physicians is infinite. If we double the number of doctors, he said, patients will make twice as many office visits.

People used to go to doctors because they were sick. Now they go because their medical insurance and a host of willing "healers" encourage them to do so. There is no doctor shortage. If only real illness were treated by physicians it would be seen that we had enough doctors to handle our medical needs—maybe too many.

II

Medical and Surgical Insurance

Some forms of surgical insurance began to appear in the 1930s. Blue Shield, the so-called doctor's plan, was established late in that decade. With huge outlays for advertising and with physicians shouting its praises, it has captured a large percentage of the surgical insurance business. Of course, Blue Shield has done much good. There is no question that in times of calamities such as serious auto accidents, severe heart attacks, or strokes, Blue Shield or any good health and accident policy is a godsend to both patient and physician.

But what of the other side of the coin? Blue Shield pays a specified amount for any of hundreds of surgical procedures. Every doctor has access to the fee schedule. Every doctor, therefore, knows ahead of time what he will get for each procedure. This guaranteed payment of fee leads to unnecessary surgery. Not only is the surgeon encouraged to operate, but the patient thinks it is not costing him anything and so he might as well get his money's worth. What the patient forgets is that every time a needless operation is performed not only does he undertake a certain amount of risk in the surgery and the anesthesia, but he also drives up the cost of the Blue Shield premiums. This has happened with sickening regularity in Pennsylvania and most other states with the result of diminished takehome pay for the Blue Shield subscriber. Note the following article:

> A unique insight into the enormous cost of health insurance is provided by figures cited by a *New York Times* article indicating that General Motors spends more money annually for Blue Shield

coverage of its employees than it pays to U.S. Steel, its major supplier of metal (The York *Dispatch,* York, Pa. August 23, 1976).

Unnecessary surgery is also one of the main reasons we constantly have to build bigger and bigger hospitals. The money needed to build these larger hospitals comes out of our taxes or from solicitation to contribute to our local hospital building fund drive. If a hospital has empty beds, hospital administrators pressure the doctors to fill up those beds. After all, the bills have to be paid on a constant overhead. But I wish to emphasize a different problem in the medical insurance system.

I have had a running battle with Blue Shield for twenty-five years. For the surgical treatment of hemorrhoids in the hospital, with surgery, anesthesia, lab work, the cost of a hospital bed, etc., the total bill is about a thousand dollars, often more. Blue Cross and Blue Shield pay the whole thousand dollars and the patient has a lot of pain and suffering and loses four to five weeks of work. For my injection treatment of hemorrhoids, in which the patient can remain ambulatory and go about his everyday business during the course of treatment, avoiding a hemorrhoidectomy and stay in the hospital, my bill is $250—but all Blue Shield will pay is $35.

If you were to have hospital surgery for a hernia or "rupture," your bills would total $1,200 to $1,500, and you would lose from eight to ten weeks of work. If I gave you injection treatment, you would have to visit my office ten to fourteen times, but you wouldn't have to stay in the hospital, and you wouldn't lose one day of work. My bill would be $350. But Blue Shield, once again, would pay only $35. For the injection treatment I perform in cases of prostatic enlargement or for any other nonsurgical method of treatment they pay nothing.

Since the success of my treatments has been documented in reputable medical journals, Blue Shield's behavior constitutes a form of discrimination against injection, or needle, surgery in the office and in favor of the costlier, very painful, and no more successful hospital surgery.

In the fall of 1971 I became so out of patience with this injustice that my lawyer and I went to Harrisburg, Pennsylvania, to see Dr.

Sydney Sinclair, president of the Medical Service Association of Pennsylvania, which administers both Blue Cross and Blue Shield. Dr. Sinclair said that he would get a review board together to consider my case. Months passed and nothing happened. After we insisted again on action, a twenty-one-man peer review was conducted, but I was not allowed to appear before the board to explain my case. The board reached their decision, and Dr. Sinclair said, in communicating it to my lawyer, that I needn't feel I was discriminated against, because four of the twenty-one men on the review board were osteopathic physicians and surgeons. Osteopaths or not, the important point is that they were all *hospital doctors*. Their decision: payment for Dr. Boyd's injection treatment remains the same. That fee was established in 1938 and was unfairly low even then. Inflation has quadrupled the cost of living since 1938, and most fees on the Blue Shield schedule have been updated several times. But the fee allowed me has stayed the same.

I then had no choice but to sue Blue Shield, which I did at the expense of several thousand dollars for legal fees. The following is a newspaper account of one phase of this litigation:

HARRISBURG, Pa. (AP)—Superior Court today was to hear a physician who charged that Blue Shield's medical plan "forces doctors to put people in the hospital" for treatment that could be performed just as effectively during an office visit.

"If Ralph Nader got hold of this plan he'd tear it apart," said Dr. Nathaniel W. Boyd III, of Loganville, York County. . . .

Boyd said Blue Shield reimburses him little or nothing for his treatments while it will pay doctors the full amount for performing surgery in a hospital to treat the same disease.

Boyd, who has treated rectal diseases for 22 years, said he uses various injection and freezing treatments to cure hernias, hemorrhoids, rectal fistulas and enlarged prostates.

"My injection treatment of enlarged prostates has been documented in the *British Journal of Surgery*," Boyd said. "In England they try to keep people out of the hospital. In this country they throw money around like water. There's no attempt to keep people out of the hospital."

Boyd, 51, said he's been fighting Blue Shield for 22 years and he gets the same answers.

"They say they don't care about me; I'm only one doctor. They say, 'Put the patients in the hospital.' I say I don't need to put them into a hospital. I've been fixing them for years in the office."

He said Blue Shield pays him $35 for his treatment of a rectal fistula using office surgery. "But they'll pay you $125 if you put the patient in the hospital, use surgery and get the same result as I did," Boyd said.

"Blue Shield is set up to aid surgeons collect money," he continued, "It's mostly a surgical plan. There's nothing wrong with that—surgeons should get paid. But why don't they set up an office schedule (rates) comparable to the hospital surgical schedule?"

We carried the case through the Commonwealth Court and the Superior Court of Pennsylvania. Both courts ruled that since I was a provider of services and not a subscriber, Blue Shield had no contractual obligation to me. In other words, my patients would have to do the suing. In my humble opinion, this was a cop-out, and if my patients had sued, these men would have found some other reason to decide in favor of city hall.

I should also mention that I am not alone in being underpaid by Blue Shield. In 1972 Pennsylvania Insurance Commissioner Herbert Denenberg held hearings in Philadelphia on the subject of medical insurance. I remember that at these hearings a number of internists complained about the inappropriate fees allowed for their work. Three or four dozen disgruntled physicians objected to the fees allowed them by Blue Shield, among them Dr. Shuman, of Philadelphia, who has successfully treated back and knee ailments with needle surgery but who has found, as I have, no fair provision for such nonhospital services in the values of the present insurance system.

Many times I have discharged patients who were very happy and satisfied until four or five weeks later, when they received their Blue Shield or Medicare check. Then they were not so happy and thought I had overcharged them, even though my fee was only one quarter of what the total fee would have been had they gone to the hospital. This type of thing makes one wonder if we really do have a free-enterprise system in this country or whether the American medical establishment refuses to allow competition to exist. Is the medical system trying to do what is best for the public? Or is it trying to do what is best for the medical system?

Medicare, the federal program of health insurance for the elderly, unfortunately uses the same fee schedules as Blue Shield, with their built-in discrimination against nonhospital treatment. When this program started in 1966 I had high hopes that finally my older patients would be allowed to have the nonsurgical treatments I performed and have most of the bill paid by the government. The plan called for a $50 deductible, the federal government picking up the tab for 80 percent of the fee that exceeded the first $50. This would have been a godsend to patients past the age of sixty-five, who constitute about seventy-five percent of my practice. But it was not to be, because the hospital doctors took control of this medical insurance system as well. The fact is that in Pennsylvania, Blue Shield administers Medicare, and in Maryland the administration of Medicare is split between Blue Shield and Travelers Insurance. Thus the same fee schedules are in effect under Medicare, favoring hospital surgery and degrading nonhospital treatment. Elderly patients who wish to stay out of the hospital for rectal, hernia, or prostate troubles must pay 80 to 90 percent of my fee out of their own pockets because hospital doctors will not reward a man for keeping patients out of the hospital.

I should explain that not all medical and surgical insurance discriminates against ambulant treatment. Some private carriers pay my fees in full; others pay a substantial part of each fee. It is primarily Blue Shield and Medicare that discriminate, but Blue Shield insures a majority of those with surgical coverage in Pennsylvania, and Medicare is all the medical insurance many elderly people have.

This is a horrible situation, but I have found that I am powerless to do anything about it. My experience in suing Blue Shield has suggested to me that we have courts of law instead of courts of justice. The judges support the hospital monopoly and do not consider the little man. A surgeon who develops new office treatment methods that work is ostracized and, as I shall detail in a later chapter, treated like a criminal.

My fees for any of my work have never exceeded one-fourth of what the total bill would have been had this same patient chosen to go to the hospital, yet hospital doctors on the fee schedule committee have the unmitigated nerve to say my fees are not reasonable and proper. What a strange world we live in! Is it any wonder I am frustrated and my patients feel that Big Brother Government does not give a damn about them?

III

Medical and Surgical Fees

What is a fair and adequate fee for a surgical procedure? This is a question with as many answers as there are people responding to it. Is $50 an hour too much to pay a skilled surgeon for performing a difficult, nerve-racking procedure? Many people who work for three or four dollars an hour would say, yes, $50 an hour is too much. Perhaps they are correct, and yet some surgical fee schedules call for much more than this for each hour of a surgeon's work.

How did surgical fees get so high? My answer is that the public, influenced by radio and television, novels, films, and the press constantly glorifying the surgeon, believe him to be some kind of superman. Few would question his fee no matter how high it was. In fact, more than a few people brag about how expensive their operations were, as if more expensive meant "better."

Another unexamined reason why surgical fees have become high is that physicians often mingle socially with wealthy people. The prestige attached to the medical profession places doctors in the same social class as the man who runs a large industrial plant employing perhaps a thousand people. I am afraid that just this association causes surgical fees to spiral higher and higher.

Such attitudes on the part of the public also help to legitimize unique advantages doctors have long held as sellers of services. A recent report, "The Problem of Rising Health Care Costs," by the White House Council on Wage and Price Stability, explains that American doctors enjoy a noncompetitive status which allows them to diagnose the ailment, prescribe the treatment, and set the price, while patients have little choice but to accept the decisions and the bills.

I do not wish to downgrade surgeons or other doctors. In general, I feel a very large majority of them are God-fearing, devoted, hardworking men who deserve respect and perhaps, like any accomplished person, a modest amount of adulation. I know of no other profession in which a man can be, and often is, called for at any hour of the day or night. But I see no earthly reason why a physician has to drive a Mercedes-Benz automobile; nor do I see any justification for his requiring that his wife be clothed in a mink coat. In truth, some exceedingly difficult surgery should be rewarded with large financial payment. The fact is, however, that routine surgery done day in and day out by a surgeon often results in a fee that far exceeds the difficulty of the task or the benefit gained by the patient.

Obstetrics is one field I can single out. Women have been having babies since time began with no aid from anyone. Of course, obstetricians will be quick to defend their sacred function by saying, "Look how much lower the mortality rate is now than it was fifty years ago." Yet the fact is that in Holland, where the infant mortality rate is the lowest in the world, 70 percent of all births are accomplished in the home without the aid of an obstetrician. The reasons we have a lower infant and maternal mortality rate now than fifty years ago are many, and most of them have little to do with the technical skill of the man who catches the baby. It is true that one case in a hundred requires specialized care. But giving birth, in general, is a normal physiological function, and far too much mumbo jumbo goes on about it. The reason the public has put up with overtreatment by obstetricians is that the gift of the new little individual placed in the mother's arms makes everything involved in the process seem all right, even the huge expense, which, by the way, is usually covered by insurance.

Another category of financial abuse includes the overuse of any new hospital surgical procedure that becomes fashionable because of its novelty.

In the middle 1960s some Japanese scientists—who were very inventive and deserve a great deal of credit—developed an instrument called a fiberoptic colonoscope. This instrument can be placed through the rectum, into the sigmoid colon, and finally advanced, in some cases, through the entire length of the large intestine, a total distance of six feet. Occasionally the tip of this instrument can even enter the terminal portion of the small intestine. This device can be manipulated by controls placed at the outlet of the rectum.

Through this instrument the physician can obtain direct visualization of the wall of the gastrointestinal tract. Photographs can be taken through the colonoscope, and some early pathologies, such as polyps, can be treated, thus avoiding an abdominal operation in some cases.

Unfortunately this procedure is being abused. People who do not need this examination at all are being forced into it. The examination is time-consuming, tedious, uncomfortable, and expensive. Surgeons are using this examination as a status symbol.

Naturally a big fee has been set up in most insurance companies to pay for this procedure. This might not be so bad if the colonoscope, which permits direct visualization, were being used in place of X rays in the gastrointestinal tract, but such is not the case. X rays are still used, and for this double service the patient is required to pay a double fee.

A doctor high up in the internal medicine department of a hospital in a good-sized midwestern city told me that his hospital hired a young physician just to do the fiberoptic colonscope examinations. The first year there he made $140,000. Unfortunately the doctor's wife did not like the Midwest, and so he left the town. What a racket his must be and how self-confident it allowed him to become! The favorable market for his fashionable specialty allowed him to walk away from a $140,000-a-year position.

Whether or not this instrument is the panacea some physicians would have us believe it is, is doubtful. Dr. William Wolfe, director of surgery at Mount Sinai School of Medicine, in New York City, warns that biopsy specimens obtained from this instrument are small, superficial, and at best random. And so it is questionable

19

whether one can be sure, for instance, whether cancer is present, even after this time-consuming and expensive test has been performed.

Dr. Malcolm Veidenheimer, chairman of the Department of Surgery at the Lahey Clinic, in Boston, declared, in the October 1975 edition of the American Cancer Society's *Cancer Journal for Clinicians,* that in cases of rectal and colon cancer, diagnosis early in the manifestation of symptoms is not necessarily diagnosis early in the course of the disease. Thus, even if the use of the fiberoptic colonoscope discovers cancer in the gastrointestinal tract, there is no assurance that the cancer will be in a stage at which treatment can be effective. If this procedure cannot benefit the afflicted patient and the physician who must treat the disease, it is of small value. And yet such a case is typical of what happens when a new type of sophisticated equipment becomes fashionable and is overused. The cost of health care escalates with little or no benefit to the public.

Once again the only possibility of a solution for this problem lies in the improvement of public knowledge. When they enter the doctor's office with a complaint, most patients do not understand what is happening to them. They feel they are in an arena of life-or-death choices and will accept any treatment the certified expert proposes and pay any fee he charges.

Finally, consider what I learned in 1971. In January of that year I met a young man of twenty-eight who was a third-year resident in psychiatry. His salary was $17,000 a year. His wife was an intern at that time, and she was making $10,000, giving the two of them a combined income two or three times as great as most families in the United States have. There was nothing here to justify that old argument that doctors should make a lot of money because they have to starve until they are thirty. These people, both still in training for their professions, were puzzling over what real estate investments to make and what stocks to buy. The high cost of hospitalization includes the cost of such salaries for interns and residents. And the high cost of treatment by physicians and surgeons includes money that we pay because our physicians and surgeons have learned while still in training that they can demand and get a high rate of pay. A few years out of school and they will expect, and get, three or four times as much.

Some physicians make over a half million dollars a year. For a physician to make over $150,000 is common. And a physician making less than $60,000 a year is considered practically a failure by his fellow doctors. But can a doctor making ten, fifteen, or twenty times as much money as his patients understand them and sympathize with their problems? Can he see things from their point of view? Can he help them decide what's best for them?

Medical Economics Magazine, sent free to all physicians twice a month, suggests that in order to retire comfortably, the doctor should have a nest egg of $500,000. Of course, the doctor should not be expected to lower his standard of living when he retires, so he will need this much to guarantee him an income of thirty or forty thousand after taxes. Well, if every doctor is going to live on an income of this size or better throughout a life of practice and in the meantime build a nest egg to see him through his retirement in the same manner, is it any wonder medical and surgical fees are so high?

IV

Osteopathic Medicine

In my twenty-eight years as an osteopathic physician I have been asked many times what an osteopath is. A fair enough question, and, I think, one that deserves an answer. At the risk of being called presumptuous by the other doctors, I am going to try to shed some light on this question. My father was a freshman at the Philadelphia College of Osteopathy in 1913, and so I have had sixty-three years of association with this fine profession, years that I hope give me the right to speak on the subject as somewhat of an expert. To my knowledge, no other doctor has gone into detail on this subject, and we cannot wait for one to do so. So here is my explanation.

The doctor of osteopathy is a fully trained physician who prescribes drugs, performs surgery, and utilizes all accepted scientific modalities to maintain and restore the health of his patients. Only D.O.'s and M.D.'s are qualified to be licensed as physicians and to practice all branches of medicine and surgery.

Today 86 percent of all D.O.'s are general practitioners, providing complete primary health care, whereas only about 25 percent of all M.D.'s are general practitioners. Over half of all D.O. general practitioners work in towns and cities with populations of less than 50,000, and in many rural communities D.O.'s are the only physicians available.

All physicians, be they M.D.'s or D.O.'s, must obtain a license from a state licensing board. For the osteopathic physician in twenty-five states the board is composed of both D.O.'s and M.D.'s, and both types of physicians must take the same examination to be licensed. In nine states licensing boards are made up entirely of M.D.'s. In the remaining sixteen states, D.O.'s alone comprise the board.

On June 14, 1971 the *Journal of the A.M.A.* showed that for the year 1970 D.O.'s who took the same medical board exam as the M.D.'s had only six failures out of 402 who took the exam, a failure rate of only 1.5 percent. The rate of failure for regular American medical school graduates was 9.3 percent, failure rate for Canadian graduates 14.0 percent, for foreign medical graduates 37.3 percent. The obvious conclusion to be drawn from this is that D.O.'s must be receiving better training.

Some 230 osteopathic hospitals located in thirty states prqvide more than 25,000 beds for treatment of the sick and injured. Colleges of osteopathic medicine receive direct financial assistance from the U.S. Department of Health, Education, and Welfare. D.O.'s are commissioned and serve as medical officers in the armed forces. Federal and state governments and public and private health agencies have recognized osteopathic medicine as a separate but equal branch of American health care. What, then, distinguishes this "equal" type of medical care?

Osteopathic medicine is a native American movement which had its beginnings in the research and observations of Andrew Taylor Still. Dr. Still was born in Lee County, Virginia, in 1828. His family emigrated to Missouri in 1837.

Having lost three children to spinal meningitis during the Civil War, Dr. Still became disillusioned with the orthodox medicine of the day. He became convinced that, to an extent, the human body is self-healing and that total bodily health depends on the proper functioning of all its systems. An unimpaired physical structure and an unimpeded flow of blood and nerve impulses to tissues are necessary, he asserted, for the systems to function properly.

Dr. Still developed a system of manipulation intended to realign abnormalities that interfered with functioning of the body's system. In 1874 he publicly proclaimed his philosophy and broke with the orthodox physicians. The U.S. Postal Service commemorated this event in 1974 with a postage stamp celebrating "100 Years of Osteopathic Medicine."

In 1892, at the age of sixty-four, Dr. Still, after many years of practicing his art, and with patients (including two U.S. Senators) coming to him from hundreds of miles away, decided to start his first school of osteopathic medicine in Kirksville, Missouri. The school and the movement grew at a rapid pace, and by the time Dr. Still died in December of 1917, eleven other schools of osteopathic medicine had been established. Six of these schools survived. But in 1962 the Los Angeles college was taken over by the medical doctors, whereupon any osteopathic physician licensed in California who elected to was given an M.D. degree if he paid a $65 fee and attended three hours of lectures a day for four weeks—a cheap way to get rid of 1,500 osteopaths.

Since 1965, four more osteopathic colleges have been started, bringing the total at this date to nine, with three more in the blueprint stage. The nine colleges presently active include the original five at Chicago, Illinois; Des Moines, Iowa; Kansas City and Kirksville, Missouri; and Philadelphia, Pennsylvania; together with the four new schools at Tulsa, Oklahoma; Fort Worth, Texas; East Lansing, Michigan; and Lewisburg, West Virginia.

The curriculum in osteopathic schools has always included all the subjects taught in other medical schools as well as courses devoted to musculoskeletal system and manipulative therapy. Since 1929 the admission requirements at osteopathic medical schools have been identical to those at allopathic medical schools (those producing M.D.'s).

The misconception exists that osteopathic practice at one time excluded the use of "medicines." One must remember that in the late nineteenth century very few drugs of a definite curative nature existed and many drugs that were in use often caused more troubles than they cured. Major surgery and obstetrics were always practiced by osteopathic physicians, and as medicines of value were developed, osteopathic physicians incorporated these into their therapeutic repertory.

The value of manipulation in musculoskeletal ailments is well known to many million open-minded laymen; the place of manipulation in the treatment of visceral disease is less well known and perhaps unknown to most people.

Physiologists, that is, men and women with doctorates in physiology (not physicians but scientists concerned with the body's physical functioning) have long known that many complicated reflexes exist. One reflex we are all familiar with is the somaticovisceral reflex, demonstrated when because our feet got cold and wet our nose runs and very often we get a sore throat. An example of a viscerosomatic reflex (one working from organ to body, rather than body to organ) occurs in the female sexual system when orgasm in the vagina, which is part of the viscera, causes flushing of the skin on the surface of the body, or soma.

There is no argument among scientifically knowledgeable people that these reflexes exist. Normalization of spinal tissues by manipulation does have an effect, through similar reflexes, on the viscera—whether the lungs, the stomach, or the arteries.

Whether manipulation was the panacea that Andrew Taylor Still thought it was is debatable, but in the late 1800s and the early years of this century, manipulation apparently cured maladies that responded to no other form of treatment then in existence. I cannot imagine any physician claiming to be a general practitioner or primary care physician who is not familiar with manipulation and trained in its use. The uses of manipulation in everyday practice are myriad, ranging from the relief of upper respiratory infections to a dramatic drop in high blood pressure. Its efficacy in musculoskeletal complaints is known to many million Americans.

Why, then, has this method of treatment fallen from favor to the point where in many communities it is difficult to get an osteopathic physician to give an osteopathic treatment? The reasons are many:

1. Manipulation is hard work. The doctor who manipulates twenty patients a day leaves his office exhausted.

2. Manipulation is time-consuming. To give three osteopathic treatments in one hour would be fast work, whereas today it is not unusual for most doctors to see six or eight or even ten patients an hour.

3. Insurance, in many cases, does not pay for manipulation,

although it often pays for other types of treatment.

4. It is easier to give medicine and forget you are a D.O.; the public does not need to be taught that pills and shots cure things, because newspapers and television constantly impress on people that this is so. But to tell a pill-oriented society that manipulation is, in some conditions, the treatment of choice is a thankless task and one which uses much of the doctor's already limited time and strength. The path of least resistance is to give pills and stop being a pioneer.

5. A small percentage of D.O.'s did not really wish to become osteopathic physicians but became D.O.'s because osteopathic physicians enjoyed a complete medical and surgical license. In addition, with the huge number of excellent students turned down for admission to allopathic medical schools each year, it is easy to see how many excellent potential physicians become osteopaths. These medical school rejects have no qualms about not practicing any manipulation, since straight medicine was what they wanted, anyway.

6. Another reason is a combination of the first, second and third reasons already given: simple economics. It takes money today to employ nurses, pay for equipment, pay the rent, pay one's malpractice insurance, and send one's children to college. Manipulators historically have never been big money earners, and after four years of college, four years of osteopathic medical school, and internship and residency, very few men are willing to settle at the bottom of the economic totem pole. If you dig into things and analyze them, it is a shame to find out how often money dominates our behavior and our actions. A wonderful form of therapy has practically been relegated to the junk pile not because it is not useful, but because it is not lucrative. I am sure the chiropractors will continue to use this fine effective form of therapy.

On several occasions I have had the unhappy experience of being at a social gathering or business conclave where an osteopathic doctor was asked by a stranger what he did for a living and hearing the doctor say "I am a surgeon" or "I am a radiologist" or "I am a doctor who specializes in internal medicine"—not one word about his being an osteopathic physician. What a complete lack of moral fiber these wealthy individuals exhibit! Here they are, existing almost totally on the referred work of the osteopathic general practitioner, the man who does the hard work of medicine, and they don't even have the decency to acknowledge that they are members of the same profession. Furthermore, here is an opportunity to let some prominent person know that we have a complete school of medicine replete with specialists in all fields, but these men lack the intestinal fortitude to stand up and be counted. These are the same men who do not want the medical doctors to take over the osteopathic profession, not because they give a damn about osteopathy but because they know that if all D.O.'s got an M.D. degree it would then be ethical for the D.O. general practitioner to send his referred work to an M.D. specialist, and the osteopathic specialist would lose much of his income.

In closing this chapter, I would like to list some of the subjects of papers presented at the scientific sessions of the North American Academy of Manipulative Medicine held in October of 1975.

1. Manipulation of the Cervical Spine
2. Manipulation of the Thoracic Spine
3. To Assess the Effect of Manipulation on Acute Low Back Pain
4. Manipulation of the Joints of the Lumbosacral Spine
5. Manipulation and the Family Physician
6. Shoulder Dysfunction Associated with Radical Mastectomy

This sounds like a list of subjects discussed at an osteopathic convention. Wrong. Every lecture was given by an M.D., and all the members of this academy are allopathic physicians, that is M.D.'s. They said we were unscientific quacks and cultists. Now, all of a sudden and very quietly, what Dr. Andrew Taylor Still said was true 100 years ago has become scientific and desirable to them.

We welcome you, doctors of medicine. Maybe we were wrong. Maybe you are not as stubborn and closed-minded as we thought you were. Come learn and absorb, and the public will be the long-term beneficiaries.

V

That Operation Is Not Necessary

WASHINGTON (UPI)—Doctors performed about 2.38 million unnecessary operations in 1974, causing 11,900 needless deaths and
costing the public nearly $4 billion, a House subcommittee said Sun-
day.

Surprised? You shouldn't be. Just about every operation ever de-
vised has been performed needlessly thousands of times, usually to
the benefit of the doctor and to the detriment of the patient. In the
United States our surgical rate per person is twice as great as the
surgical rate in countries where doctors get the same pay no matter
how many operations they perform. The American doctor's motive
for much of this surgery is greed, and sometimes more than one
physician is involved. In some places a kickback system exists
through which the general practitioner gets a percentage of the fee
on all the surgical work he sends to the hospital. This condition has
existed and has been denied for years, but my experience leaves me
with no question that it still goes on in many localities. It is much
more likely to go on where there is an excess of surgeons and few
general practitioners. The surgical work then goes to the highest
bidder, the general practitioners, who spread their referrals
around, ending up, in some cases, with a higher total income than
any of the surgeons.

Physicians, I believe, have an unparalleled opportunity to do
good for their fellow man, and part of their pay should be the
satisfaction of helping other human beings. I would much rather
talk about the amount of surgery I have prevented than the amount

of surgery I have been forced to perform. Any good confidence man with hospital surgical privileges can do a great deal of surgery and capture huge fees. But is this really why we became doctors? If the aim is to become wealthy, why not be a businessman?

Not all unnecessary surgery is the physician's fault; some patients have an overwhelming and compelling desire to have surgery performed. A typical case is that of the wife whose husband is not paying as much attention to her as he did fifteen or twenty years ago. An operation will, for a little while at least, put her back on center stage in the attention of her family and friends. Paradoxically, this needless surgery sometimes temporarily clears up all of the patient's symptoms, which were of a psychosomatic nature in the first place.

But it is usually doctors, rather than patients, who advocate unnecessary surgery; and their motivation is, as I have said, often financial. Sometimes, however, it is ignorance, and not greed, that is responsible for needless operations, doctor as well as patient being unaware of the alternatives to surgery. In the chapters following this one I will discuss specific techniques, little known by doctors and still less known by the public, which permit the successful treatment of hernias and rectal and prostate ailments without hospital surgery. In this chapter I will survey briefly a few other areas in which unnecessary operations and other hospital procedures are all too common.

Tonsillectomy

How many of you still have your tonsils? Chances are at least four to one that if yours are out they should not be. In the back of everyone's throat at birth is some lymphoid tissue called Waldeyer's ring. One of the lymphoid structures included in Waldeyer's ring is a pair of small organs called tonsils. They were not put there to be taken out indiscriminately at six or seven years of age. This tissue fights infection, although it sometimes swells and results in sore throats. Occasionally tonsils should come out, but tonsil removal should never have become a routine procedure.

In the 1920s and 1930s the old-time osteopath spoke out against the routine tonsillectomy and was laughed at and scorned by most medical men. But in the 1940s and 1950s, when the osteopaths began to build their own hospitals, they started to yank out tonsils without hesitation. To talk against tonsillectomy during this time was medical heresy.

Today the ear, nose, and throat specialists are publishing papers saying that tonsils should stay in. The persecuted osteopaths of fifty years ago apparently were right in the first place. But unfortunately tonsils still are coming out at a far too rapid rate. According to one study, about 500,000 needless tonsillectomies are performed each year in this country. Experience even shows this operation occasionally results in death. Not long ago, a prominent family in my community lost a child during this operation.

Appendectomy

Among the medical men I have known, I remember well a man who would rush patients into the hospital, usually late at night, so that he could operate immediately on their appendices. Bringing the patient in at night, he was able to go ahead with surgery he claimed was "a matter of life or death," without routine lab procedures available to confirm or deny his diagnosis. This man was commonly referred to as "Hot Belly Harry" because an acute appendix is called a "hot belly."

One day a patient he had hauled into the hospital vomited, and the pain in his belly soon went away. The patient had only had an upset stomach and no appendicitis at all. We can only wonder how many others of Hot Belly Harry's appendectomy patients were in a similar situation but had their appendices needlessly removed. And we can wonder how many other Hot Belly Harrys there are in our hospitals.

Hospitals have tissue committees that are responsible for guarding against unnecessary surgery. These committees examine organs and tissue removed from the body in surgery to assure that the tissue was not normal and should have been removed. However, in the case of the appendix, this does little good, because, as pathologists have informed me, virtually any appendix in a person past age fifteen will show, on microscopic examination, chronic recurrent appendicitis. That means that most of us sometime in our lives have had a bellyache that probably was a mild attack of appendicitis. But we did not need, and many people who have lost their appendices did not need, an appendectomy. Figures show that 4 of every 1,000 people who undergo an appendectomy do not survive the surgery.

Hysterectomy

The hysterectomy, or the removal of the uterus, has frequently been called the "rape of the abdomen" because most doctors have acknowledged that it is done too often and needlessly. In some cases of cancer, removal of the uterus is lifesaving, and in most cases of cancer it prolongs life. The most common reason for removal of the uterus, however, is endometriosis, or the overgrowth of normal tissue in abnormal locations within the uterus, ovaries, or urinary system. This excess tissue causes abnormal bleeding, which robs the woman of strength ("blood-loss anemia") and sometimes becomes severe enough to make necessary the removal of the uterus.

The needless removal of the uterus, however, I believe, is criminal. It often gives the patient a barrel-shaped abdomen and results in the loss of feminine characteristics, for instance, through the growth of excess body hair. Many women have also told me that sexual sensitivity in the genital area was greatly diminished for them after they had had this operation. Even with female hormone shots and pills these symptoms sometimes persist. One should remember that every operation carries some risk of unexpected problems. Death may occur, and just surviving the operation can mean pain and suffering. Unsightly scars on the body, infections picked up in the hospital, headaches after spinal anesthesia, the general debility and feeling of weakness that almost always follows major surgery are just some of the problems. According to a recently completed Cornell University study, 260,000 unnecessary hysterectomies are performed in the United States each year.

Cholecystectomy

Another operation that is performed too often is the cholecystectomy, or the removal of the gall bladder. We hear all the time about the wonderful progress medicine has made in the last fifty years, and it is true that some of this new knowledge, if properly applied to diseases such as those of the gall bladder, will eliminate much needless surgery.

The routine removal of the gall bladder when gallstones are found on a patient's X-ray should certainly be condemned. At least fifteen million Americans have gallstones, and most of them are symptom-free.

In younger people thirty to fifty years of age, the death rate in the hands of the very best surgeons doing elective cholecystectomies is only one tenth of one percent—about as low a mortality figure as can be found in any type of major surgery. After the age of sixty-five, however, the mortality rate rises to between 4 and 5 percent—a high death rate. The physician has at his disposal various medicines that will dilate the hepatic duct, the cystic duct, and the common bile duct and relax the spincter of Oddi, where the bile is let into the small intestine. Dilation makes passage of the bile easier and alleviates pain. In addition to these valuable medicines, drugs are available that do a good job of liquifying the bile, thus making the gall bladder function better and helping to prevent stasis and the formation of gallstones.

If the patient under fifty finds little relief of symptoms and no diminution of the pathology after a good solid try with the above methods of treatment, then—and only then—surgery is definitely indicated. If the patient has developed gall bladder problems after the age of fifty, then because of the increased risk of death and the increased risk of other sequelae that accompany all surgery (nausea and vomiting, headache from spinal anesthesia, etc.) then the operation should be avoided.

A nonsurgical method for the dissolving of gallstones with the use of chenodeoxycholic acid has recently been reported by Leslie Schoenfield, M.D., director of gastroenterology at the Cedars of Lebanon Mount-Sinai Medical Center in Los Angeles and director of the National Cooperative Gall Stone Survey. This new medicine has been used in at least six hundred cases in the United States, Europe, and South America and has completely or partially dissolved gallstones in 70 percent of the patients. Unfavorable side effects from the medicine were few. Diarrhea did develop in 20 percent of the patients, but this stopped when the dose of cheno acid was reduced. Some of the patients were followed for two years after the dissolving of their stones, and in only 10 percent of these cases was there a recurrence of the stones. This implies that in cases of recurrence some form of continuing prophylactic therapy may be indicated, perhaps a low daily dose given every day of the week for one week each month.

The cost of the chenodeoxycholic acid is today about a dollar a day. Since treatment is necessary for only a couple of months and then probably can be terminated, this treatment would seem quite cheap compared to surgery. Cheno acid has at least shown that the dissolving of gallstones is medically possible.

Kidney Stones and Urinary Bladder Stones

Surgery for kidney stones and urinary bladder stones, or renal calculi as they are technically named, should also diminish as new treatments that replace or at least limit surgery are developed. The Commission on Hospital Activities estimates that 38,000 Americans undergo surgery each year for the removal of kidney stones and 14,000 are operated on for the removal of urinary bladder stones.

Two new drugs said to prevent kidney stones are allopurinol, which is used in the treatment of gout to prevent formation of uric acid, and the antihypertensive diuretic trichlormethiazide. A seven-year study of 202 patients was made and the patients' rate of kidney stone formation during drug therapy was found to be almost 90 percent below what it had been before treatment. The side effects were minimal. Skin reactions (in 3 patients) and rising alkaline phosphatase levels (in 2 patients) disappeared with the discontinuation of allopurinol.

Dr. Alex Raney, a top urologist and chief of urology at the Veterans' Administration Hospital in Wilmington, Delaware, states that a new electronic device in the form of a thin metal probe that sends out pulsating shock waves at the rate of 100 per minute has successfully pulverized stones in 90 percent of the cases in which he has used it. This procedure does require, in the case of the kidney, that the body be cut open so that the kidney can be reached, but cutting into the kidney, probably the most dangerous operation in urological surgery because of the chances of complications and even death, can now be eliminated. In the case of stones in the urinary bladder, the probe can be inserted through the urethra, thus eliminating surgery completely.

For kidney stones a short stay in the hospital is needed, but it is usually one half the stay required after the nephrolithotomy, the cutting operation on the kidney. Patients with bladder stones can be treated on an outpatient basis, or at worst must go into the hospital for three days.

This valuable work is also being done by Dr. Irving Bush, chairman of the urology department at a Chicago medical school, whose results corroborate those of Dr. Raney.

Laminectomy

Another very debilitating surgical operation is the laminectomy, or the removal of a herniated disc anywhere in the spinal column. I am much encouraged by the attitude of some of the younger orthopedic surgeons who seem to realize that many back operations are simply not succeeding and that more conservative management of these conditions is warranted. Again, I do not wish to leave the impression that surgery is never indicated; in properly selected cases disc removal results are dramatic. Disc problems and their treatment will be discussed more specifically in a later chapter.

To eliminate unnecessary surgery one should always get a second and even a third opinion. Do not go for the second opinion to a doctor who is a member of the same medical group as the first surgeon consulted. Do not even tell the second or third doctor that you have been told you need surgery. Today conformity has become such a ritual that we have all too appropriately been labeled a nation of sheep. Few people today, and this includes doctors, do much thinking for themselves. If you tell the second or third doctor that surgery has already been suggested, he doubtless will think to himself, "Who am I to disagree with Dr. X? Besides, this person already has surgery on his mind." I am not trying to imply that most surgeons are knife-happy, but they are human beings; and if the patient already is half-sold on surgery, the job of convincing them that they need surgery is made very easy.

Some of the most high-caliber men I have ever had the pleasure of knowing were surgical specialists, and they deserve a great deal of respect and recognition. Many surgeons are men of integrity; so if not one but three surgeons independently decide that you need surgery, then go ahead—and good luck.

A word about other hospital specialists is needed. I was once told by a certified radiologist (an X-ray specialist) that if he took a million X-rays and discovered only one case of cancer that was otherwise unsuspected, the expense of the million X-rays would be justified. This is the type of fuzzy thinking that has driven the cost of doctors and hospitals out of sight. Who pays for this overutilization of laboratory tests? You do, John Q. Public. I do not feel the medical profession has the means or the guts to police this kind of abuse. In fact, the problem may well not have a solution.

The public has been so brainwashed about laboratory testing that even in cases of hemorrhoids, which I have never known to contain cancerous material, patients sometimes demand biopsies to test for cancer when the experienced physician knows that such biopsies are unnecessary and a waste of laboratory facilities and the patient's money.

The question of laboratory testing brings us to another type of needless cost associated with surgery. The results of many of the lab tests both patients and physicians demand are all too often wrong. Senator Edward Kennedy recently announced a National Bureau of Standards finding: 26 percent of the laboratory work done in Medicare-reimbursed labs was either false or incorrect. For example, patients go through the trauma of being told that they have cancer when actually they do not. Or their minds are put at ease when told they do not have cancer or some other serious disease, and they learn later, sometimes on their deathbeds, that they did have cancer all along.

Studies indicate that bad laboratory performance is demonstrated by 20 percent of laboratories in bacteriological testing and 40 percent in simple clinical chemical tests. Even in blood typing and blood grouping the errors ran up to 18 percent. One study has shown that in a screening procedure for a type of female cancer either suspicious cells were overlooked or a cancer was wrongly reported 30 percent of the time. It is such waste and misuse of facilities and such overutilization of tests, I am convinced, that drive up the cost of hospitalization. The truth is that in some cities the average hospital charge per day is now over $115, three times as much as it was only twenty years ago. With hospital costs so high, there can be little doubt that if there were no Blue Cross and Blue Shield and no doctors willing to prescribe hospitalization to get for themselves and their hospitals the guaranteed fees, over 50 percent of the beds in America's hospitals would be empty.

Medicaid for the poor and Medicare for senior citizens have been abused in ways similar to the ways Blue Cross and Blue Shield are taken advantage of. The quick-buck artists, whether owners of laboratories or unscrupulous physicians, apparently have discovered that this is the golden road to wealth—financed by your tax money and mine. I do not know why controls have not been set up to stop this senseless waste of our resources. Occasional news articles are published about a doctor's being indicted for alleged Medicare fraud, usually for $50,000 or more. I know the smaller robberies of our tax money are not prosecuted. A "deal" is commonly made, and the thief who has gotten money for services he never performed, or for performing surgery on people who do not need it, thereby escapes public scrutiny. The crime of the surgeon who willfully performs surgery on people who do not need it in order to get a guaranteed fee is especially grievous. He not only steals public money, but he puts some unsuspecting patient through an ordeal that accomplishes nothing but the lining of the doctor's pockets.

If physicians were honest and devoted to their patients' well-being instead of their own convenience and enrichment, much unnecessary surgery and laboratory testing might be replaced or forestalled by the careful history taking and thorough physical examination that used to be the rule. The physician of the "old school" used all five senses to make the diagnosis—sight, hearing, touch, smell, and even (because these men were more dedicated than most modern doctors) taste (doctors used to taste the patient's urine in diagnosing diabetes).

Today, under the guise of better health care, the patient is subjected to such a battery of laboratory tests that one wonders why the doctor spent twelve years past high school in training. Why not put everything in a computer and come up with a diagnosis? Why have doctors at all? Why not just have technicians to interpret the results of the tests? Laboratory tests to confirm a diagnosis are helpful, but it does not take much of a doctor to order a thousand dollars' worth of tests. These are some of the chief reasons our hospital bills have gotten too high and monthly insurance premiums are difficult to meet.

But not only lab work and surgery are overprescribed. We are also dangerous overusers of medicines. A beloved Johns Hopkins Medical School professor, Sir William Osler, is quoted as having said, "If all the medicine in the world were thrown in the ocean, it would be worse for the fish and better for the people." The number of sleeping pills and tranquilizers being gulped down every day in this country is almost astronomical, and it is a sad tribute to our current lifestyle.

Proper attention to a well-balanced diet, regular exercise, and adequate sleep and relaxation would eliminate some of this useless and increasing drugging of the public with sleeping pills. Sleeping pills should never be used on a permanent basis, although occasionally they will solve a temporary problem with no significant bad effects. Tranquilizers, on the other hand, are a greater hoax perpetrated on the public. People pop them into their mouths like candy, and, like candy, they solve nothing. Doctors are taught in school to treat the causes of disease. I know of no disease that was ever caused by low tranquilizer levels in the human body.

On a more personal note, I will confess that when I was past forty years of age I started to drink coffee for the first time. I know that I now have certain minor problems with my health that, I am sure, are caused by the coffee, but I am hooked. When I drink it I temporarily feel good; nevertheless I know that this temporary euphoric feeling is not worth the price the human body pays for it.

Instead of a coffee break twice a day, every day, all people, regardless of age, should have an exercise break. This exercise should be of a nature appropriate to one's age, weight, and physical condition.

The founder of osteopathic medicine, Andrew Taylor Still, said over a hundred years ago, "The rule of the artery is supreme." He meant by this that adequate, complete circulation of the blood through the body would enhance the well-being of any patient. What could be better than sensible, vigorous exercise, enough to raise the pulse rate fifty to sixty beats a minute, for fifteen minutes, twice each day. Most adults seldom use more than half of their lungs' capacity; that is, they rarely fill their lungs completely with air. Vigorous exercise—enough to cause you to pant—will force you to inhale and exhale fully and thus get fresh oxygen-carrying air to all parts of the lungs. The heart will be strengthened, and will push more blood with each contraction. The elasticity of the arteries will thus improve, possibly preventing heart attacks and strokes.

And stop smoking. The connection between smoking and cancer and heart and great vessel disease can no longer be denied. And there is another harmful effect of smoking which has received no publicity. It involves the substance in our blood called hemoglobin, the red pigment that carries oxygen to all the living tissue in our bodies. Carbon monoxide is released when tobacco is burned, and you and I get the effect of it, whether it is we who smoke the cigarette or somebody else.

The CO we breathe in combines chemically with our hemoglobin to form carboxyhemoglobin in our blood, a substance which thwarts the true function of hemoglobin. This compound does not take up and give off oxygen during the circulation of our blood and acts as an asphyxiant. Carboxyhemoglobin is a very stable compound, and it takes many days of breathing fresh air to completely eliminate it from the system. In the meantime the symptoms of its presence, familiar among garage mechanics, who breathe carbon monoxide from car exhausts, may appear, subtle but damaging: chronic tiredness, lack of pep, and recurrent headaches. There is another side to Dr. Still's rule of the artery: good health does depend upon good circulation; so if the blood's ability to transport oxygen is damaged, general bodily health will be damaged, too.

Skepticism about the practices of modern physicians and hospitals can help you to avoid unnecessary surgery and laboratory testing. But it should go without saying that the best way to avoid surgery and medical expenses is to remain healthy. It has been said that healthy exercise can add years to your life. Whether that is true or not, exercise will certainly add *life* to your *years* and decrease the likelihood of your needing any kind of medical or surgical treatment.

VI

Rectal Disease

Rectal disease must be nearly as old as man himself. Rectal diseases are numerous, hemorrhoids being by far the most common, and the history of the treatment of hemorrhoids goes back many hundreds of years. Ancient treatments included cauterizing with a hot iron and various methods of surgical removal. These methods were, of course, very painful and often left the patient with a scar on the rectal wall at each operative site and a rectum so narrow that pencil-sized stools were the rule. The patients often wondered if they had not been better off in their original condition.

In 1871 Dr. Milton W. Mitchell was practicing his profession in Clinton, Illinois. He was not very busy, but he did have as patients a few old farmers with "piles," or hemorrhoids. Dr. Mitchell experimented with the injection of various solutions and fluids into the pile mass and finally came up with a solution that stopped all bleeding and rectal protrusion. This method of treatment was taught to other doctors who were interested in rectal diseases and handed down through the years to doctors who either had no hospital facilities or were opposed to putting their patients through the hell of a surgical hemorrhoidectomy. The hospital surgeons, of course, immediately opposed this unorthodox treatment. They were being made to look bad by the lowly general practitioner turned proctologist.

In those early days around the turn of the twentieth century, there were two things legitimate rectal specialists had to contend with. The first was that hospital specialists saw a threat to their monopoly in the elimination of the need for the surgeon, the anaesthesiologist, the X-ray specialist, the pathologist, and the specialist in internal medicine in dealing with rectal problems. The second was that some men, some of whom were not even physicians, tried to practice the injection treatment of hemorrhoids just to make a fast dollar. These men, who had no real interest in helping sick people, did not really learn how to do the work properly, and their sloppy results, achieved through poor efforts, brought condemnation not on themselves but on the method of treatment.

Of course, with 99 percent of the medical profession against the method of treatment to start with, failures were magnified and quickly talked about throughout the medical community. Without Establishment acceptance, no formal standards or training period were established for this work. The only way to learn it was to go to another physician's office and watch him do it.

In 1929, Dr. Frank D. Stanton established the Dover Clinic in Boston, Massachusetts, to teach the ambulatory treatment of rectal diseases (literally, treatment in which the patient can keep walking; treatment which does not require confinement in the hospital). From that date until 1958, when the clinic closed, Dr. Stanton and his staff trained over five hundred men to do this work. Unfortunately for the public, most of these men had hospital affiliations and soon became hospital surgical proctologists and turned their backs on the injection method. Why did this happen? Again, there were two reasons. First, if the patients had any question after treatment in the hospital, the doctor was not disturbed—the nurse down the hall took care of it. Secondly, that old thief of our freedom of choice, surgical insurance, reared its ugly head and for some strange reason decided that the doctor's fee in the hospital should be five or six times as much as the doctor's fee in the office. Naturally, doctors, being human, put their patients in the hospital so that the nurse could handle the problems while they (the doctors) were "insured" a liberal reward for their work. Once again the doctor's convenience was satisfied instead of the patient's needs. The insurance companies' fee schedule committees, made up of hospital specialists, by allowing a very small fee for nonhospital

41

treatment, have forced the patient into the hospital, thus filling a hospital bed and providing work, and, of course, fees, for numerous auxiliary specialists and laboratory technicians.

Anatomy

There is probably no part of the human body so little studied as the anal-rectal region. There is also no part of the body in which the average physician has less interest. I have known excellent physicians who, when asked by a patient to look at their rectum, dodged this part of the body as if touching it would cause leprosy.

The rectum is a muscular pouch extending from the top of the anal canal to the sigmoid flexure of the large intestine. This tube or pouch is movable and varies in size and condition in different individuals. This area contains Houston's valves, which probably tell our brain when we should go to the toilet.

Hemorrhoids occur in the lower portion of the rectum and in the anal canal, below it. The anal canal is separated from the rectum by the pectinate line (Hilton's Line), as shown in figure 1. Above this line there are no pain fibers, and this is why most hemorrhoids can be treated absolutely without pain by the injection method. Internal hemorrhoids above the pectinate line are best for the injection treatment, but when hemorrhoids extend from the rectum into the anal canal (internal and external hemorrhoids), results below the line can be had from injection above the line. Below this line the pain can be exquisite, as anyone who has ever had real trouble in this area knows.

At the level of Hilton's line lie the rectal crypts, varying in number from five to seven. These crypts are supposedly there to secrete a small amount of lubricant to ease the passage of fecal matter. These anal-rectal crypts of Morgagni are the seat of the infection in anal-rectal fissure and fistula, after hemorrhoids two of the most common rectal complaints men and women are heir to. By the way, the huge difference in the width and length of the anal-rectal canal accounts for some individuals' being able to move more fecal mat-

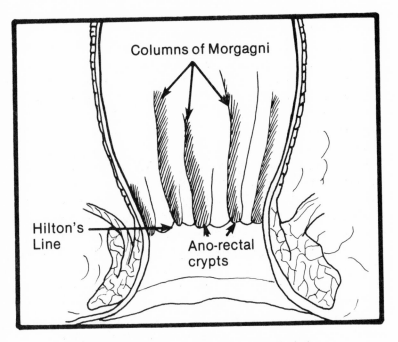

Fig. 1. Terminal four inches of anal-rectal canal.

ter out in one bowel movement than other persons can in four or five bowel movements.

The blood supply of the rectum is made up of the hemorrhoidal plexus of veins, some two hundred in number. These veins enter the rectum in the greatest numbers in three areas: the right anterior, the right posterior, and the left midline. It is in these three areas that 98 percent of all hemorrhoids develop. The function of these veins, besides supplying the rectum with blood, is to absorb water, making the fecal mass smaller and more solid so that the rectal muscles can do their job and keep us from soiling our clothes. I could write another ten pages easily on the anatomy of this area, but in relation to rectal diseases most of the salient points have been covered thoroughly enough to help the lay reader understand what is to follow.

Hemorrhoids are probably the most common ailment of a continuing nature known to man. At times they seem to improve with no treatment, but they usually return worse than before. Many preparations and salves are sold for the relief of the symptoms of hemorrhoids, although little of a permanent value generally is gained from their use.

The causes of hemorrhoids are probably several. Mankind's upright position has frequently been blamed—in other words, gravity is the offender. This is probably a factor, yet many four-legged animals suffer from hemorrhoids. I personally think that many severe bouts of constipation and diarrhea can be a cause. Pure hemorrhoids, most proctologists agree, usually have their start in infancy or even at birth, the disposition to develop them being inherited. According to this theory, hemorrhoids result from a congenital excess of tissue in the lining of the anal-rectal canal. Strain of one sort or another causes this excess lining to be pulled loose from the canal wall and form "piles" or hemorrhoids. The symptoms of piles are bleeding (usually the blood is bright red), protrusion (if they are bad enough), and often a full, dragging feeling inside the rectum.

In the most common form of hemorrhoids the mucous membrane lining has been torn loose from the muscular wall of the rectum. (Figure 2.) This normal lining of the rectum can be cut off, and the average surgeon will do this if given half a chance, because he does not know any better. In many cases, however, structural integrity can be maintained by injecting a substance which has a sclerosing nature from which complete relief can be obtained in as few as three or four treatments—if a skilled needle surgeon is in charge of the patient. Figure 3 shows the technique of injecting hemorrhoids.

A judicious injection of the correct scleroising agent, used in the right place, in the right quantity, and at the right time, will give these people excellent therapeutic results. This form of cure works like the injection of a powerful wallpaper paste beneath paper

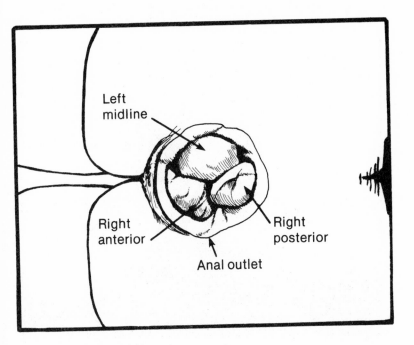

Left
midline

Right
anterior

Right
posterior

Anal outlet

Fig. 2. The three primary hemorrhoidal masses.

hanging loosely from a wall. The sclerosing solution creates fibrous tissues which draws the wallpaperlike tissue strongly back to a flat position against the wall of the rectum. The normal structure of the anal-rectal canal is restablished, and normal functioning in this area is thus restored without cutting away any part of the body. Such treatment is in accord with the thinking of Dr. Andrew Taylor Still, whose dictum "Structure governs function" implies that treatments are to be preferred which reestablish, rather than alter, the original structure to the organism.

But the injection of hemorrhoids cannot be done by handing a needle and syringe to a surgeon and saying "Here, go ahead." It takes years of thoughtful experience to become proficient in this work.

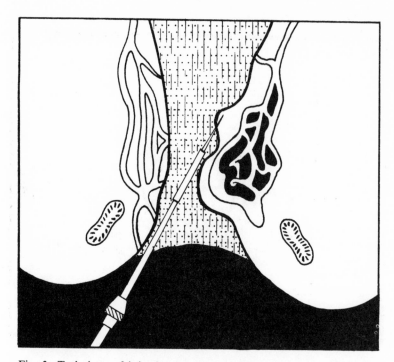

Fig. 3. Technique of injecting hemorrhoids. The injection is placed beneath the mucous membrane lining of the rectum.

I have been asked many times, "Do hemorrhoids become cancerous?" The answer is no. The two conditions are distinctly different phenomena. However, it is possible to have hemorrhoids and carcinoma at the same time.

Hemorrhoids, besides being an embarrassment (with their discomfort, itching, and soiling of clothes), can cause anemia of a chronic nature because of a considerable blood loss that occurs perhaps daily over months and even years of time. This undetected anemia can cause headaches, fatigue, a loss of appetite, and a lack of energy.

There are many different kinds of hemorrhoids and patients will experience varying types and degrees of symptoms. But all can be treated in the office, generally without surgery. This is not to say that occasionally a small amount of cutting with local anesthesia is not needed to achieve a better cosmetic result.

Anal-Rectal Abscess and Fistula

Any boil or accumulation of pus within three inches of the anal opening has to be considered an anal-rectal abscess until proven otherwise. If the doctor finds that the abscess communicates with the rectum as soon as he opens it, it becomes a fistula. An anal-rectal fistula, simply stated, is really a tunnel that starts with an infection at the crypt in the anal canal, the pus formed there burrowing its way under the tissues and following the path of least resistance until it forms a pool of pus under the skin. Opening this abscess, or fistula, gives quick partial relief (and abscesses often break open spontaneously), but the abscess will recur if surgery is not properly done. This surgery involves the insertion of a metal probe through the drained cavity and through the fistulous tract communicating with the infected rectal crypt. An incision is then made through the rectal wall to completely open the fistula, which then heals quite easily.

Anal-Rectal Fissure

A fissure is, as its name indicates, a split or tear in the mucous membrane of the anal canal. Figure 4 shows the external appearance of a fissure. This painful condition can be cured 100 percent of the time by the ambulant proctologist, and often he can cure it without any cutting at all. Local anesthesia is injected, and the physician, by stretching the relaxed anesthetized anal sphincter with his well-trained fingers, performs finger surgery, which loosens the spasm in the area, breaks up adhesions, and reestablishes normal circulation in the rectum. In about two weeks the rectum becomes, through the body's own self-curative power,

47

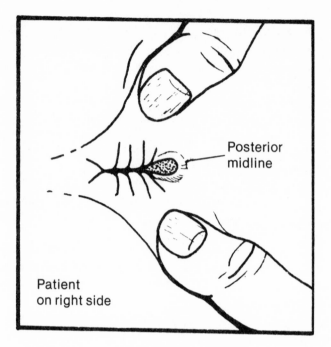

Fig. 4. Fissure.

symptom-free and healed. The rule of the artery is once again supreme: with the reestablishment of normal circulation the body begins to heal itself.

Rectal Symptoms

Bleeding, pain, and itch (or burning) are the most common symptoms of rectal disease, the signs by which hemorrhoids, an abscess, a fistula, a fissure, and other conditions make themselves known.

Bleeding. Bleeding from the rectum is the most common of rectal symptoms. To assume that the blood is from hemorrhoids can be a serious mistake. Bleeding that is expelled at the beginning of the

48

bowel movement usually comes from hemorrhoids. Blood, however, that is seen late in the bowel movement usually comes from a higher part of the anal-rectal tract and probably is more serious.

It is wrong to assume that all bright red blood comes from the lower part of the rectum and that all dark or black blood comes from a higher part. Blood from the lower part of the rectum can be retained for a long time and be very dark when expelled. Blood in conjunction with getting up in the middle of the night to move the bowels, gripping pain, passing a lot of gas, mucus, and a bowel movement of a not very normal consistency, is possibly a sign of rectal cancer and should quickly send one to a physician.

Pain. Sharp pain in the rectum brings a patient to the proctologist in a hurry. He or she may have had rectal itching or bleeding for years and have more or less ignored it, but if he really starts to hurt he comes running. To the physician, bleeding and a change of bowel habits are the most serious rectal complaints but pain is number one to the patient.

The pain of an anal rectal fissure is typically a sharp and deep cutting pain on bowel movement, which, when very bad, can bring tears to the eyes of the most stoic of strong men.

The pain of an abscess and eventual fistula is gradual in its development, and is usually accompanied by swelling and, eventually, symptoms of general sickness throughout the body. Fever is common, and nausea, a loss of appetite, and an elevated white blood count may occur. An anal-rectal abscess has the greatest systemic effect of any of the ailments treated by the ambulatory proctologist.

Another cause of rectal pain is "clot piles," hard little lumps caused by the obstruction of one or more small veins. These can easily be removed in the office.

The dull throbbing pain of rectal protrusion is great, especially if the sphincter contracts after a large hemorrhoidal mass has been pushed out. Besides internal hemorrhoids, hypertrophied papillae may protrude, or the protrusion may be an external thrombotic hemorrhoid. Whereas internal hemorrhoids may be simply replaced in the rectum and then treated by injection, the external thrombotic hemorrhoid must first be opened and the blue-black clotted blood at its center removed. This is done under local anesthesia in about five minutes. Unnecessary hospitalization for this problem has been known to waste three days of a patient's time in the hospital and ten days away from work.

Itching. In my practice the third most common presenting symptom of anal-rectal patients, after bleeding and pain, is itching and burning around the anal outlet. The causes are myriad. *Pruritus ani,* or rectal itch, is rarely a local disease but is generally connected with deeper causes, such as diet or a fungus infection. A notable exception is contact dermatitis, caused by washing with a soap to which the patient is allergic. Underpants washed in detergent that the patient cannot tolerate or the development of a fungus infection caused at least in part by not enough air getting at that part of the body are possible causes of rectal itch. Almost all cases of rectal itch would be greatly helped if the patient removed his pants three or four times a day and let an electric fan blow on the anal-rectal area for ten minutes at a distance of one foot. A dry perianal region is usually an itch-free perianal region.

My considered opinion is that the large majority of rectal-itch sufferers have a diet that causes most of their troubles. First, go easy on condiments: pepper, horseradish, garlic, and potent relish items like scallions, radishes, and pickles. You should avoid, as well, smoked foods and highly seasoned sausages, scrapple, and so forth. Second, beware of citrus fruits and citrus juices, which can cause an alkalinity around the anal outlet in which fungus infections love to dwell. Instead, if you have rectal itch, drink moderate amounts of cranberry, grape, and prune juice to regain normal acidity. Third, keep away from white sugar and white flour. Use brown sugar and honey if you feel you must eat sweets. Chocolate can also cause rectal itch. Switch to whole wheat bread. Spaghetti, macaroni, pizza, and pot pie can be offenders. In other words, use your head and stop eating junk. Eat plain, simple fresh or frozen meats and vegetables. They are better for your general health as well. Of course, not all rectal itch and burning are caused by diet. Some rectal diseases can cause itch—protruding piles certainly can, and anal fissures can cause itching as well as pain. An anal abscess or fistula certainly can cause burning and pain.

Whatever the origin of their symptoms, most rectal-itch sufferers can be completely cured non-surgically. A small amount of judicious surgery done in the office under local anesthesia is occasionally needed in cases in which itch has been present for years and a lot of daily scratching has taken place, but I will make this statement categorically: no rectal sufferer whose primary complaint is rectal itch will get complete, permanent relief by going into the hospital and having a general surgeon perform a surgical procedure on his rectum—unless this physician is well read, has a real interest in rectal diseases, and goes over in detail with the patient his diet and many of the other things I have just mentioned.

Pilonidal Sinus

During the war a pilonidal sinus was often called "jeeps disease." Actually, the bumping up and down in jeeps only stirred up and activated a condition that had been there since birth. *Pilo* is a Greek word meaning "hair." *Nidal* is a Greek word meaning "nest." Thus a pilonidal sinus, or pilonidal cyst, is literally a hair nest. This condition is caused by an embryological defect which causes the products of the ectoderm to be buried instead of on the surface of the body.

The presence of a pilonidal sinus is indicated by the appearance of one or two (or as many as twelve) small holes between the tailbone and a point about three inches upward toward the patient's low back. The holes are not necessarily on the midline, but the hair nest is always located along the midline. The skin may have a gray discoloration around the holes, from which hairs may protrude. These holes are sometimes quiescent, but if bumped or struck they are likely to become actively painful and begin to produce the pus or watery discharge typical of this condition.

Office surgery is satisfactory in curing pilonidal sinus. An incision is made in the midline, and the hair and other products of the ectoderm are completely removed from beneath the skin.

Condylomata Acuminata

Condyloma Acuminata is a condition that causes a rectal protrusion which can grow to a very large size. It looks like a mass of cauliflowerlike warts and is fairly common. It is called *condyloma acuminata* and can be easily fixed in the office with local anesthesia and clean surgery. Little bleeding occurs and pain is minimal, but the surgeon must be sure he gets all of the grapelike masses or the condition will recur.

Condyloma acuminata is also known as genital warts and can occur on the lips of the vagina and anywhere on the male penis as well as in the anal region. In the anal region their presence indicates that a penis with genital warts has been in your patient's rectum.

Hirschsprung's Disease

Another condition the proctologist sees, but for which there is unfortunately not much in the way of a cure, either ambulatory or in the hospital, is Hirschsprung's disease, an illness in which the lower part of the large intestine is found to be greatly dilated in a baby at the time of birth. Hirschsprung's disease is a congenital malady and occurs chiefly in the male child.

Along with dilation of the large intestine (from which the disease gets its other name, congenital megacolon) there seems to be an imbalance in the nerves of the intestinal wall, which results in the brain's being unable to tell the large intestine to empty itself. In some cases bowel movements are as infrequent as every several weeks, and, as might be expected, when a stool is finally passed it has an extremely bad odor. In other cases the young boy never has a bowel movement on his own, and enemas must be given daily or three times a week.

In a bad case the child will remain thin and the outline of the entire large intestine will be clearly visible through the abdominal wall. Even when the outline of the intestine is not visible, the abdomen is enlarged. The diagnosis of Hirschsprung's disease is easy to make from this characteristic potbelly and the almost complete lack of voluntary bowel movement in a very young child.

The medical treatment of this condition is usually not satisfactory, and enemas are rarely completely eliminated. Some authorities claim to have a degree of success with surgery, usually through the cutting of nerves such as the presacral nerve. Such treatment may help the patient, but the permanent sexual impotence that this operation produces in the male child is definitely a major consequence to be considered.

Constipation

A physician friend of mine, an excellent proctologist and needle surgeon who taught me a great deal, Dr. R. L. Capers, of Bellefonte, Pennsylvania, who died in May 1976, said to me many years ago, "Doctor, to be a success you only have to be able to do one thing—learn to cure constipation." What is constipation? The simplest definition is the inability to pass a stool of normal consistency as often as is necessary. How often is necessary? I have had patients who only had three or four movements a week, but I would not say they were constipated, because the movement was not hard or dry.

To prevent constipation drink at least twelve eight-ounce glasses of fluid a day. Fruits and vegetables should be in the diet, because roughage always helps maintain moisture in the gastrointestinal tract. Avoid foods that you know from experience constipate you, such as nuts, milk chocolate, etc. Always eat breakfast, and eat foods of a bulky nature, that is, of a fibrous nature—cereal or a slice of whole wheat bread. The word "breakfast" means break your overnight fast. Eating a sensible breakfast will stimulate persistalsis of the entire gastrointestinal tract. Establish a habitual time, after breakfast perhaps, to go to the toilet and sit, taking your time, knees up. Place a footstool by the toilet and place your feet on the stool; have your knees higher than your hips, and go to the toilet at the same time every day.

Most human beings have what we doctors call a gastrocolic reflex. This means that if a large, bulky, wet mass of food is ingested, reflexly a peristaltic wave is set up that pushes the food along the intestinal tract, thus pushing the previous meals' food ahead of it, like one railroad freight car pushing the car ahead of it along the track. This results in a desire to defecate. The problem with most laxatives is that they knock two or three cars off the track at one time, and then there is no bowel movement for two days because nothing is there.

Adequate exercise is also important in preventing constipation. Sit-ups are especially helpful. Having someone hold your ankles to the ground. This exercise increases the intestinal tone.

My favorite non-habit-forming laxative, if you wish to call it a laxative, is metamucil, a powder which holds water in the fecal mass until it leaves the body twelve to thirty-six hours after being swallowed.

Many times constipated people do not eat enough fats. Because of all the publicity given to cholesterol in recent years, I have actually seen people go overboard and not eat enough oil and fats. Oleomargarine will provide some oil of an unsaturated nature and will not raise the cholesterol level but will help prevent constipation. Bulky foods give the gastrointestinal tract the type of material needed to stimulate peristalsis.

Diarrhea

Diarrhea is usually due to the ingestion of some food that does not agree with one, and the condition is self-limiting, usually ending within forty-eight hours. Minor diarrhea can also occur when one is under some nervous strain. This will clear up when the nervousness is removed.

Loose bowels can occur, along with rectal itch, if an antibiotic is used to treat an upper respiratory infection. Such medicine is a mixed blessing. It often eliminates the infection, but it often kills many friendly bacteria in the intestines. These bacteria, of the acidophilus group, must be replaced before normal bowel movements can resume. Any diarrhea that gets out of control should be treated immediately, because dehydration can rapidly ensue and the electrolytic balance can be thrown off. This can lead to serious systemic disease.

Loose bowels caused by certain organisms are not diarrhea but dysentery. They can be extremely dangerous and occasionally lead to death even with the best methods of treatment. Visitors to Mexico occasionally become ill with dysentery that does not respond even to heroic measures, and deaths from this cause have occurred among tourists in Mexico as well as elsewhere.

Anesthesia for Rectal Diseases

The one thing patients dread most is pain. Fortunately today we have ointments available containing local anesthetics that the rectal specialist can apply with his finger to the painful rectal area before attempting an examination. The wise use of these preparations makes most rectal examinations almost painless.

As I have previously stated, the injection treatment of piles or hemorrhoids should be painless. The needle should be inserted in the area above the pectinate line, where no pain fibers are present. If the patient desires surgery, or if a condition is present requiring surgery, this presents no problem to the experienced ambulatory proctologist.

The introduction of local anesthetics to the surgical scene was one of the greatest achievements of the late 1800s. I have seen gall bladders and appendices taken out under local anesthesia as well as hernia repairs done with such anesthetic. I have never seen a bad reaction or a complication from the use of any modern local anesthetic. Most of the problems occurring in the hospital operating room are not the effects of surgery but the results of complications involving general anesthesia.

Because all, or nearly all, hemorrhoidal tissue is eliminated with the painless injection treatment, very little surgery is required for hemorrhoids. Anesthesia for any surgery that is necessary may be obtained by first using a very small needle and a few drops of a local anesthetic just under the skin to make a "wheal," or numb area, on the surface. This prick might be felt for five seconds. Anesthesia of the entire rectum can then be completed through the wheal, with no additional pain to the patient. I know this is hard to believe, but patients often remark, "If I had known it would hurt this little, I would have had this done twenty years ago."

Neglect causes progression of disease. The patient who is apprehensive and fearful causes problems for himself and his physician by his delay.

VII

Hernia

A hernia is a protrusion of any viscera or tissue through an abnormal opening from the cavity in which it is normally confined. The term *rupture* is generally used by the public to designate abdominal protrusions, but this term should probably be discarded because it properly infers a breaking or tearing through the muscles, and this practically never happens. Hernia is almost always due to a birth defect which provides a potential opening through which the viscera later protrude. This does not mean that a hernia is present at birth. The defect is there at birth, but the hernia may not show up for many years.

Hernia is one of the more common major conditions affecting mankind. Probably 6 percent to 8 percent of male adults have had, have, or will have a hernia sometime in their life. Many women also develop hernias. There are many types of hernias, the most common occurring in the groin, low and far to the side; this type, called inguinal, accounts for 92 percent of all hernias. Other common hernias are umbilical (or navel) hernias and femoral (in the thigh) hernia. Inguinal hernia occurs nine times more often in men than in women, while femoral hernia, a far less common ailment, occurs three times as often in women as in men. Figure 5 shows the locations of the common types of hernias. Statistics show that 25 percent of all hernia sufferers will give a history of hernia in their parents or grandparents. I have often treated grandfather, father, and son for hernia, and 75 percent of the time my records show the hernias occurred on the same side of the body.

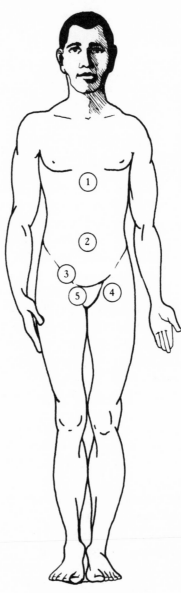

1 Epigastric.
2 Umbilical.
3 Inguinal.
4 Femoral.
5 Scrotal.

Fig. 5. Types of hernia.

There is definitely a hereditary factor involved, but that is not to say that events during the life of the individual play little or no part. It has been noted before that the operation for the removal of the appendix can create a disposition toward hernia. Inguinal hernias are generally 10 percent more likely to be found on the right side of the abdomen than the left side. In patients who have had an appendectomy, however, herniation is 25 percent more likely on the right side, where the appendectomy incision is made, than on the left. Dr. Leigh Watson explains that this phenomenon results either from injury to the iliohypogastric nerve during the appendectomy or from failure to close the transversalis fascia properly at the end of the operation. "Structure governs function," as Dr. Andrew Taylor Still, founder of osteopathic medicine, insisted. Interference with the normal structure of the body during an appendectomy, which might have been unnecessary in the first place, can sometimes lead to a breakdown in normal functioning and eventual herniation.

Hernia is undoubtedly as old as man. It was probably treated by primitive man with the simple measures at hand, guided by his instinct. As knowledge increased, reducible hernia—in which the protruding intestinal contents may be pushed back into the abdominal cavity—was retained by a girdle, the forerunner of our modern truss. Strangulated hernia—in which viscera are clamped on by the inguinal ring, through which they protrude, and are thus not able to slide back into the abdominal cavity—was treated by a light diet, rest, purgatives, and the application of cold water or snow to reduce swelling. Massage and inverted position sometimes helped return the abdominal contents to the abdominal cavity, where they belonged. While the earliest records of surgery go back to the year 4000 B.C., in Mesopotamia, the first recorded surgery for hernia was in the first century A.D. Celsus, a Roman, operated on quite a few hernias at this time. The modern surgical treatment for hernia dates back to the introduction of antiseptic surgery by Lister in 1871.

My treatment for hernia, the nonsurgical or injection treatment, originated in 1832, when a Dr. Jaynes, of St. Louis, started to use it. In 1835, Velpeau, of France, also started to do the work in a small way. The first really prominent man to do a great deal of this work was Dr. George Heaton, of Alton, Illinois. Heaton was graduated from the University of Pennsylvania Medical School in 1831. He then went to Boston, Massachusetts, to practice his profession. After several years of the successful treatment of hernia by the injection method, with his theories and claims supported by case histories and hundreds of cured patients, Heaton invited the representatives of the medical profession in Boston to see him perform the injection. His invitation was declined because it was considered an act of impudence, and he never again made such an offer in this country.

The newspapers advocated his cause and directed public sentiment in his favor. Dr. Heaton from then on enjoyed even greater success. Having once been refused a reception by his profession, he continued to keep secret both his technique and the composition of his injection solutions in reaction to this jealous and spiteful treatment by American doctors. Medical writers seem to agree that Dr. George Heaton, between 1831 and 1879, actually cured more patients of reducible hernia by the injection method than had been cured by all methods up to this time.

In 1845 Heaton visited London, where he was made a member of the Royal Chirurgical Society, the Westminister Society, and The Royal London Society. Heaton was then invited to Paris, where he was similarly honored. He enjoyed a large and lucrative practice in Boston, continually at odds with the members of his profession but well thought of by the public. Heaton died in the year 1881, a genius who had cured several thousand people of hernia, guilty only of never having performed an unnecessary operation, and probably having saved several dozens of lives by avoiding surgery. The medical profession in the United States looked down its nose at him for forty-eight years. This is the price the renegade must pay, but as Harry Truman once said, "If you can't stand the heat, get out of the kitchen." I must say that today very few doctors can stand the heat of the kitchen. They avoid this distinguished and successful form of treatment for no good reason.

Inguinal Hernias Suitable for Treatment by Injection

I am often asked which hernias are suitable for treatment by this method. The best one-sentence answer I can give—and I shall call it "Boyd's Law"—is this: *Any hernia that can be held in place with the middle three fingers of one hand while the patient is standing on his feet is suitable to be treated by the injection method.*

Older people are excellent candidates for this treatment because they build up fibrous tissue faster than young people and they are not as apt to do extremely heavy work after a cure has been effected as younger people are. In addition, older people are worse hospital-surgical risks than young people. One out of every four hernias I treat has already had hospital surgery, a fact which leads me to believe that the recurrence rate with hospital surgery is much higher than the surgeons admit. I believe the best surgeons would be found to have a failure rate of 10 percent if their cases were followed for five years. Those patients who have had surgery do not usually return to their surgeons and inform them of recurrences. They tell me, "Why should I go back and tell him? I certainly do not want to go through that again." At my clinic we treat some of these surgical failures, but our cure rate for them is not over 70 percent. These patients also experience more pain from injections than fresh cases.

The Surgeon General of the United States Army announced on April 23, 1942, the following policy of his office concerning waiver for limited service officers. I quote from Section 2: "The following may be recommended for general military service with waiver. . . . (G.) History of operation or of injection treatment for inguinal hernia, provided examination three months following operation or the last injection shows a satisfactory result." Despite such recognition of the injection treatment, it is amazing how the natural conservatism of the average physician causes him to condemn a method of which he has no direct knowledge. I can recall a patient of mine asking a medical doctor, now dead, who practiced twenty miles from me, what he thought of Dr. Boyd. He answered, "The damn quack!" Then he took a breath and probably because he was basically a fair man, said, "But he sure has fixed a lot of hernias."

61

I can recall another patient's asking another physician what he thought of his going to me to have his hernia fixed. The good doctor said, "I don't believe in it." Then he said, "But how can you argue with him? He has been doing the work successfully for a quarter of a century." In other words, he acted as if it were a religion.

What makes my treatment work? I often tell my patients, "It is like chopping wood. At first you will get a blister on your hand from the irritation of the axe handle against your skin, but if you stick with it you will eventually build up a thick callus on your hand." The injection treatment of hernia effects a cure by the same mechanism. A solution is injected which causes a build-up of fibrous tissue. Instead of fibrous tissue buildup on the hands, the fibrous tissue buildup is in the inguinal canal and tightens the internal and external inguinal rings and disposes of the hernial sac by retaining it within the newly strengthened wall. One does not inject the hernia; one injects the rings and the canal through which the herniation travels toward the man's scrotum.

Treatment of a hernia of course begins with a very careful history. The doctor first examines the patient while the patient stands without a truss on. Then the doctor reduces the hernia and examines the hernia with the patient flat on his back. The surgeon then fits a good padded and leather-covered steel hood truss on the patient, which must be worn night and day during the entire course of treatment. The patient is treated at weekly intervals, the patient always lying flat on his back and his feet raised, his head and shoulders lower than his legs. The patient will feel a slight pinprick with each treatment; but only for a second; the rest of the treatment is practically painless. After each treatment some slight pain is felt intermittently for twenty-four to forty-eight hours. Mild pain pills, of course, may be taken; and ice placed over the injection site off and on the day of treatment can be of help, but seldom is it needed.

Loss of time from employment during the treatment of a hernia is practically unheard of, but care must be taken. The patient should take sponge baths, since getting in and out of a bathtub without a truss would interfere with the fibrous tissue formation.

After all, one does not take a cast off a broken arm while the arm is healing. With the wise use of lamb's wool and an automobile chamois, the truss can be made comfortable.

The treatments are given at one-week intervals for the first ten treatments and at two-week intervals for the last four treatments, a total of approximately fourteen treatments during eighteen weeks, during which time the truss, of course, must be worn. This schedule varies with the size and nature of each hernia. Occasionally a patient finds it convenient to come in once every three weeks, but the truss must then be worn for a longer period. When the truss is permanently discarded, any reasonable activity that was engaged in previous to the onset of the hernia can be resumed. A hospital bill is saved, no ugly scar is left on the belly, no time is lost from work, and pain and suffering are minimal.

Of course, the medical insurance company usually makes only a token payment because the fee schedule committees of all insurance companies are made up of hospital specialists. This is one of the evils of the system which we have already explored, one of the reasons the poor citizen no longer has control of his own body. Many of my would-be patients, with tears in their eyes, say, "Doctor, if I go to the hospital my insurance pays everything, but if I come to you I pay almost all of the bill." The implication is also there, although unspoken, "If your treatment is any good, why will the insurance not pay for it?"

What doctor is going to use his time, his brain, and his ingenuity to develop new office treatment methods if the medical Establishment refuses to pay for them? If the insurance industry can continue to force doctors to put people in the hospital, there will be no end in sight: hospitals will get bigger and more expensive every year. Is it any wonder that we are rapidly drifting into government control of medicine? *Doctors, through their greed and selfishness, will kill the goose that laid the golden egg.*

Indications for Injection Treatment of Hernia

The vast majority of people who have hernias—about 85 percent—can be permanently helped by the nonconfining and practically painless injection treatment. This includes a huge number of people who would never submit to surgery, but would wear a truss forever, so great is their fear of the knife. Most of these patients tolerate injection treatment very well.

People who have health problems that would make surgery difficult, such as high blood pressure, heart trouble, kidney problems, and diabetes, all make suitable patients. Diabetics can be treated for hernia by the injection method with complete safety.

People who cannot afford surgical and hospital insurance and certainly cannot bear the prohibitive cost of hospitalization and surgery out of their own pockets find injection treatment appropriate for them.

Then there is that group of sufferers who for religious reasons refuse blood transfusions or surgery but who accept this treatment gladly.

This treatment does not upset routine. Patients can be treated on their way to work, on their lunch hour, or on the way home from work, even if they face a long streetcar ride or an hour or more in an automobile. Older people past the age of sixty, seventy, or even eighty tolerate this kind of treatment well.

Not only does this treatment save money, but it saves a lot of time, and patients are not required to stay away from home, family, or job.

Instructions for Patients Being Treated
For Hernia by the Injection Method

The proper wearing of the truss is as important to the cure of a hernia as is the skill of the doctor. One would not take the cast off of a broken arm every night to see how one's arm was healing, because this would break up the newly formed bone tissue. One can just as surely break up the newly formed tissue healing one's hernia if one takes the truss off every night to check one's progress.

Only sponge baths can be taken. Sitting down in a tub or standing in a shower certainly will break down newly formed and inadequately firm new tissue. The truss cannot be worn during baths or showers, because long exposure to water would rot its leather covering.

After ten to twelve treatments the truss can be taken off for sleep. Patients often ask if they can take two treatments a week or three treatments a week and dispense with the truss after six weeks. The answer is no. The injections produce a residual soreness in the belly which it is best not to enter soon again with the needle. An exception might be made in the case of unusually stoic patients who could stand treatments more frequently than once a week. Even if the injections were hastened, however, the truss would still have to be worn for six weeks after the final injection. We have done research on this and know by microscopic examination that it takes six to eight weeks for each treatment to adequately build up firm strong tissue. So, naturally, six weeks must elapse after the final injection to derive the full benefit from all treatments.

If you develop a bad cough within six months of being treated, put the truss back on until the cough goes away.

Doctors Trained in This Work

Unfortunately, the medical hierarchy has decided it is not in their best interests to establish any type of training program in this work.

My one-man efforts have been laughed at and scorned. I have been made to feel that my work is somehow unclean and that I should have my mouth washed out with soap. My early training in this work consisted for the most part in getting the information out of the few books written on the subject and watching a few doctors give the injections in their offices.

I also took all the work I could get dissecting bodies in the areas of my interest from those practically nonexistent men who had a cadaver or two and who taught me anatomy in private. The anatomy learned in medical school is not sufficient to enable a physician to do this work. It is amazing how the fingertips of the hands can be trained to feel through one to two inches of skin, fat, or fascia (connective tissue). As a little trick, I have often shown friends how I can feel a piece of string through 300 pages of a telephone book. The injection method has been criticized as a blind procedure. The degree to which it is blind depends largely on the surgeon's anatomical knowledge and his ability to feel and know what he is feeling.

Femoral and Umbilical Hernia

Femoral and umbilical hernias can also be treated by this method, although there is less call for such treatment because these types of hernia are far less numerous than the inguinal type. Naturally a different type of truss must be used, but it is worn, of course, for the duration of the treatment. Figure 6 shows the method of injecting an umbilical hernia.

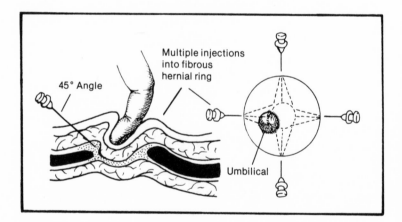

Fig. 6. A method of injecting an umbilical hernia.

66

I do not treat umbilical hernias that measure over three quarters of an inch in diameter, and they must be freely reducible. Usually these cases require fewer treatments and a shorter period with the truss than do inguinal hernias.

Hiatal Hernia

I am often asked whether a hiatal hernia can be treated by injection. The answer is no. A diaphragmatic hernia, or hiatal hernia, is a protrusion of the stomach up into the thoracic or chest cavity through the hiatus, or opening in the diaphragm through which the esophagus enters the abdominal cavity. It is often associated with poor muscle tone and/or obesity. This fat and poor muscle tone tends to push the abdominal contents through the hiatus in the diaphragm. The diagnosis is made by X ray. The pronounced symptom is heartburn, since acid from the stomach is refluxed into the gullet. The repair of the hiatal hernia is a formidable operation, and it is frequently performed unnecessarily. The basic treatment, if the patient is too heavy, is to lose weight, take antacids, and diet by taking frequent but smaller meals.

Finding a hiatal hernia on an X ray is not reason enough for surgery. It must be ascertained that the symptoms are truly due to a hernia, because some stomach ulcers and gall bladder dysfunctions will give the same symptoms. The repair of hiatal hernia is rarely needed if the patient is given the correct medical treatment.

In conclusion, I would like to dispel a myth and offer a word of advice to anyone who finds himself with a hernia.

Living near York, Pennsylvania, as I do, being friendly with Mr. Robert (Bob) Hoffman, owner of the York Barbell Company and publisher of *Strength and Health Magazine,* and being a former athlete, I have spent some time lifting weights and have watched much weight lifting. Bob Hoffman has been for many years the United States Olympic weight-lifting coach and is a real authority on this sport. In my conversations with Mr. Hoffman he has said that he never knew of a trained weightlifter who had acquired a hernia from lifting weights. Thus it is that industry in general does not look kindly on claims that hernias were acquired at work. Before the year 1880 the English courts correctly held that traumatic hernia could occur only from direct violence resulting in a definite tearing of the abdominal wall. All other hernias were considered due to birth defects.

If, because of the action of strain on a weakness present since birth, one should find oneself with a hernia, one should immediately be fitted with a good steel truss, which should be worn night and day if possible. I have seen hernias that were so large and came out with such a propulsive force that I strongly doubt that the best hernia surgeon in the country could permanently repair them by any means. Most of these hernias began very small, but neglect and stupidity made them so large that the individual became practically an invalid.

VIII

Rectal Disease—For Doctors

When the new patient with a rectal problem walks into the office, first take a good searching history. Be most careful to ask all questions that will help determine the possibility of cancer. It does absolutely no good to cure the hemorrhoids, the fissure, the fistula, etc., if cancer is present just above the reach of the examining finger.

For the examination, have the patient lie down on his right side, his knees drawn up on his chest, the left knee slightly more flexed than the right knee. First examine the skin of the perianal area, making sure there are no external fistulous openings. Also notice whether the patient has done any scratching. Many times it is found that a patient who does not complain of itch has been scratching the area around the anal outlet. Upon further questioning the patient will admit that, yes, it does itch occasionally. The chief complaint was so much more severe that he did not bother to mention the itch. Be sure, however, to keep your patient happy by treating all symptoms present, even the itch, which might be a minor symptom. After scrutinizing this area carefully, insert a well-lubricated index finger, covered by a finger cot, slowly into the rectum. Be careful; this is a sensitive area.

Now examine the tone of the sphincter anti-externus. Is the muscle in spasm? Is a fissure present? Is the patient overly nervous? Often the patient will bear down even though no real problem is present in this area. In men, slide your finger anteriorly until it touches the prostate gland. Is the gland normal in size? If enlarged, is the consistency normal? Remember that cancer of the prostate occurs most often in the part of the gland that can be palpated through the rectum. Then advance your finger deeper until it is inserted fully. Feel for a tumor of any type; a carcinoma feels like a piece of uncooked cauliflower. Remember again that 50 percent of all cancer of the sigmoid colon and rectum is within reach of the examining finger. Very often it is, however, barely within reach. Therefore, reach in very deep. Of course, a history of getting up at night to move one's bowels or a change in bowel habits, such as alternating diarrhea and constipation, is very often pathognomonic of cancer.

Notice when you withdraw your finger whether any blood is present, and if so, what color it is. Is it mixed with stool? If your patient has any stool in his rectum, is it hard, dry, or soft? With cancer the blood usually has a characteristic watery appearance. The odor of cancer of the rectum is distinctive, hard to describe, but once smelled, not easily forgotten. Make sure no abscess is present. Remember that a rectal abscess starts at the crypts but may move toward the head. If this happens, a soft bulge will be felt with your finger in the rectum. It is possible in some cases of abscess to have a patient who is quite sick with a low-grade fever to rather high-grade fever with apparently no rectal symptoms. Finding and opening such an abscess will immediately give blessed relief to the poor sufferer and make him think you are a saint. In making a diagnosis, you must first, and above all, be suspicious.

If a painful fissure or stenosis is present, do not perform a speculum examination until you have administered local anesthesia. I find lidocaine 1 percent to be an excellent local anesthesthetic. I give orally one and one-half grains of sodium pentobarbital or three grains if the patient drinks much whiskey or beer, one-half hour before administering the local anesthetic. Give the lidocaine (½ cc), with a twenty-four-gauge one-inch needle, superficially, usually in the posterior midline, to create a wheal. Allowing about three minutes for the initial injection to take effect, switch to a twenty-gauge two-inch needle and, with your left index finger in the rectum, inject through the wheal, with your right hand, up to 20 cc of lidocaine to thoroughly anesthetize the area. This amount will be sufficient for any surgical procedure on the rectum that is performed through the rectum. This, of course, does not include abdomino-perineal resection for cancer, etc., when the belly also has to be opened. The average patient will seldom complain.

If more than 20 cc of the anesthetic is needed, your technique is faulty. Huge amounts of anesthetic injected because of lack of expertise cause 99 percent of all anesthetic reactions. Local anesthetics are almost without side effects. What a pity they cannot be used for all types of surgery!

We then proceed to the speculum examination of the rectum. This is done, of course, without anesthesia unless some very painful conditions makes anesthesia necessary. Slowly insert a well-lubricated and warmed speculum. Examine the crypts of Morgagni and the papillae. Make sure the crypts are not infected and the papillae are not enlarged. Examine the rectal mucosa. Does it bulge or is it pendulous? Is it normal in appearance? No blood or mucous discharge? Have the patient bear down. Often this presents some mass above the reach of the examining speculum.

When you have finished this examination you should decide on a course of treatment. If possible, the spouse of the patient should be present during the examination and join in a discussion concerning treatment. It is most valuable to obtain the cooperation of those around the patient at home.

Injection Treatment of Hemorrhoids

If the diagnosis is hemorrhoids, first decide how complicated they are. Nearly all hemorrhoids can be greatly helped without any cutting of any type. In fact, many can be completely cured by the painless method of needle surgery. If you decide to treat the patient by the injection method, the technique follows. Remember, much practice is needed to acquire excellence in this work. It is not to be taken lightly. Hundreds of injections must be given before you

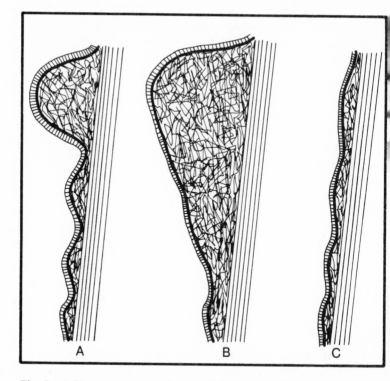

Fig. 7. a) The mucuous membrane of the rectum pulled away from the muscular coat of the rectum. b) Appearance of mucuous membrane immediately after injection, showing distention caused by the volume of the injected fluid. c) Appearance of same site one week later, showing how the mucuous membrane lining of rectum is drawn taut, cemented against the muscular coat of the rectum.

really know what you are doing. When perfected, however, you have a marvelous tool at your disposal. Unfortunately, to my knowledge the injection technique is not being taught today in any medical school. Instead, so much surgery is being taught that this method is becoming a lost art.

To begin, the doctor must tease the hemorrhoid into a Barr-Shufford speculum, using a metal probe, until as much as possible falls into view. Leave the speculum in the rectum for two minutes or more before starting the injection. This allows more hemorrhoidal tissue to enter the speculum, as a result of which more fluid can then be injected and a better result can be obtained. The needle should penetrate the mucosa over the hemorrhoidal mass. Then lift with your needle to be sure you are not in the muscular wall of the rectum—the needle tip must be freely movable.

How much do you inject? You inject whatever the tissues will take, whether 1 cc or 20 cc. Yes, 20 cc. This is the problem of critics of this method of treatment who claim to have tried it without success: they did not inject enough fluid.

A very well known New York proctologist who published a book on ambulatory proctology in 1946 and has reedited his book at least twice states in his chapter on the injection treatment of hemorrhoids that the treatment is of value in *some* cases. The good doctor, whom I have met several times and who certainly is a pleasant enough gentleman, then goes on to describe his technique, stating that he uses a 2 cc syringe and a dose of 2 cc—of course, with this size syringe a larger dose would be impossible. If this man only uses a dose of 2 cc, then I can easily see that his injections are of only limited value and understand why he has turned to the surgical treatment of his hemorrhoid patients. I have seen in medical textbooks recommended dosages of ½ cc or ¼ cc of injection fluid. This amount will never do the job. Critics of this method who purport to have tried it and found it lacking probably also had cause for failure in the weakness of their sclerosing solution and in their insufficient knowledge of where and how to properly inject it.

As you inject, look for the striation sign (so named by Charles Elton Blanchard, M.D., now deceased, of Youngstown, Ohio). This striation sign is an appearance of lines that become more distinct on the walls of the mucosa as you inject. This striation is due to the superficial vessels of the mucosa showing as red lines. From experience you will learn just when to stop injecting the solution. If a white spot appears, you are not deep enough—stop the injection immediately. To continue could cause bleeding.

When finished, always massage the area with your finger to spread the medicine around under the membrane. Hemorrhoids grow in three main areas: the right anterior, the right posterior, and the left midline. Be sure to look closely in these three areas for hemorrhoidal tissue. Always treat them with as much solution as the tissues will take. Three huge doses will do far more good than the same amount of medicine injected in fifteen or twenty smaller doses. However, the insurance companies pay a fee of so much per office visit, thus encouraging a doctor who is less than honest to treat a patient fifteen or twenty times to get the maximum amount of money the insurance allows. Such payments clearly indicate that the insurance companies do not understand how the treatment works.

If the doctor yields to this inducement, his patient ends up with a worse result, while the patient's expenses are, of course, tripled. So if a doctor knows how to do the work and does it in four office visits, he and his patient are penalized, while the inept doctor, who, because of lack of expertise, needs three times as many treatments to get a less satisfactory result, will be paid three times as much money.

Any patient with hemorrhoids suitable for treatment by the injection method can be cured in no more than five office visits.

How the Treatment Works

What does the injection accomplish? By inducing adhesion to form as a result of the chemical irritation of our injection solution, thus establishing natural support for the hemorrhoidal plexis by firming up the interstitial and adventitial tissues, we have restored the rectal mucosa to its normal tonicity and thus have removed all redundancy.

74

Limitations of the Treatment

There are occasional cases in which protrusion has been present for so many years that the sphincter has shut down on the protruding mass. This may cause strangulated thrombotic hemorrhoids. The external hemorrhoids may be covered by true skin. In such cases the hemorrhoids are best removed by simple surgery, using local anesthesia and sharp scissors, in the office. If the incision is carried above the pectinate line, ligatures should be placed at the cephalic end of the incision to assure hemostasis. This is easily done under local anesthesia in the office.

Injection Solution

The injection solution consists of a strong sclerosing agent I prepare from readily available materials.

Fissure

Probably the second most common rectal complaint is the rectal fissure. Fissures occur at the pectinate line in the posterior midline 95 percent of the time. Occasionally they occur in the anterior midline in women, but rarely at this location in men. They hardly ever occur at any other location. The nonsurgical treatment of an anal-rectal fissure is a divulsion done under local anesthesia with the index fingers of both hands inserted into the rectum about one to two inches. Patients do not complain when this procedure is used with properly administered anesthesia. The physician stretches the external sphincter. After performing a dozen or so of these operations, on learns just how much force to use. Be sure to stretch it enough; it is difficult to overdo. No patient has ever accused me of causing him to lose bowel control, no matter what procedure I have performed. In 90 percent of the fissures or anal-rectal stenosis, a divulsion will do the job. In a very bad, long-standing case, office surgery is sometimes needed and easily accomplished. Establish total rectal anesthesia at the posterior midline, and using a Bard-Parker knife or a Cosmo cautery unit, cut through the subcutaneous portion of the sphincter ani-externus. This maneuver will heal a fissure no matter what its location. You have broken up the muscle spasm, and healing will take place from the bottom up.

Anal-Rectal Fistula

A fistula is a tunnel or passageway created when an anal-rectal crypt becomes infected because of a fishbone or some other hard, dry material (such as a poorly digested piece of corn) or perhaps because of a forceful bowel movement containing some hard, dry material. This passageway starts in a rectal crypt and opens up somewhere out on the buttock or posterior thigh. Dr. Frederick Salmon, an English surgeon who died in 1859, left a body of knowledge about the treatment of fistulas that many hospital surgeons still do not know. At least 90 percent of all external fistula openings are within one inch of the anal verge, and Salmon's Rule states that the canal in these cases goes directly into the nearest crypt, wheel-spoke fashion. Salmon's line is a line drawn through the rectum, between the right and left ischial tuberosities, thus dividing the rectum into equal anterior and posterior halves. (Figure 8).

Salmon's Law states that if the tract of any fistula which upon examination has an external opening anterior to this line upon palpation if the tract is found to cross this line, then its internal opening will be found in the posterior midline crypt. This knowledge will prevent much needless cutting, cutting that would not cure the patient. In doing fistula surgery, never go around corners and never make angular incisions. Simple fistulas, those that go straight into the rectum (see figure 9), are easily fixed by any good surgeon. The more complicated fistulas, those whose external openings are over one inch from the anal verge, are best treated with respect. Radical surgery done in one stage can easily lead to

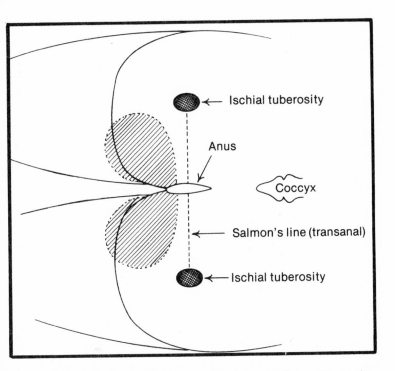

Fig. 8. Salmon's line, dividing the rectum into anterior and posterior portions.

deformity of the anal outlet and possible incontinence. Remember that a fistula always heals toward its internal opening. With this in mind, I feel, in a difficult case a cautious approach is warranted.

Cut along the inserted metal probe toward the internal opening. Do not make a curving incision; stay straight. Stop when you feel you can go no further without tempting deformity. At this point I like to put in place a waxed thread seton (a piece of thread that will not disintegrate). Thread it through the channel from the internal opening to the rectal end of your incision. Leave this seton in place for three weeks. Complete the operation three weeks later. Occasionally a three-stage operation is wise; it takes longer but gives you the assurance that the patient's sphincter will remain func-

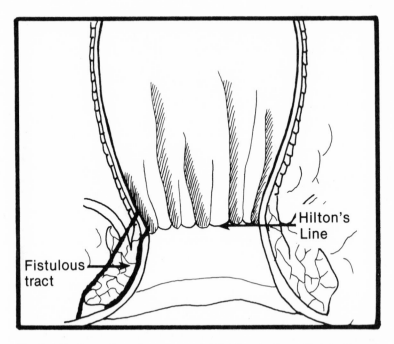

Fistulous tract

Hilton's Line

Fig. 9. The formation of an ano-rectal fistula, starting with infection of a crypt, pus burrowing under pressure until it breaks out through the skin of the buttocks.

tional. Patients who even partially lose control of their bowels are never in a very forgiving mood.

Sphincterotomy

In surgical procedures performed in the area of the anal-rectal outlet the ambulatory proctologist sometimes cuts muscle tissue. He never cuts the internal sphincter muscle, but he sometimes cuts part of the external sphincter.

The external anal sphincter muscle is made up of three parts: the profundis, superficialis, and subcutaneous parts. The doctor never

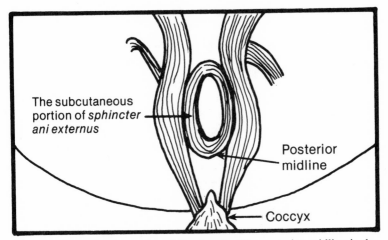

The subcutaneous portion of *sphincter ani externus*

Posterior midline

Coccyx

Fig. 10. The perineal muscles of the female. The posterior midline is the point where muscle is cut after hemorrhoidectomy and in ano-rectal fissures.

cuts the profundis or the superficialis part of this muscle; he very often cuts the subcutaneous part. In doing fistula surgery, he usually does. In fissure surgery and in hemorrhoid surgery he always does.

As you can see on the anatomical illustration, figure 10, the subcutaneous portion of the external sphincter encircles the outlet like a purse string. Like a purse string, it tightens to restrict and hold the contents within or loosens to allow the contents out. This muscle is cut for three important reasons:

1. To prevent postoperative pain. Pain following rectal surgery occurs because this muscle, made up of striated muscle fibers, goes into spasm and thus seriously interferes with the flow of blood. Once again, as A. T. Still proclaimed in 1874, ''The rule of the artery is supreme.'' When the circulation is interfered with, healing is slowed and pain results. When the fibers of the subcutaneous part of the muscle are cut, spasm is stopped, pain is minimized, and healing ensues. The cutting of this muscle is one of the reasons our patients have so little pain after surgery.

2. To prevent postoperative stenosis, or narrowing, of the rectum which results in pencil-thin stools. When the subcutaneous muscle is cut, the wound site stays relaxed for ten days to two weeks, during which time a great deal of healing takes place. When the muscle fibers reunite, we have a normal, good-sized rectal outlet instead of a narrow, stiff, and frozen one.

3. To prevent fecal impactions. A fecal impaction is a piling up of stool in the anal canal, and I think it is obvious that cutting this muscle would help prevent such an occurrence. In twenty-six years of proctological surgery I have had one fecal impaction. One day in mid-November 1952 I decided I would do a hemorrhoidectomy without doing the sphincterotomy that (as Dr. Stanton taught me at the Dover Clinc) we always must do. One week later I regretted my rashness. I found that pulling out a pound of fecal matter from a patient's rectum with one's index finger and an iced-tea spoon takes at least fifteen minutes, during which time the patient is in considerable pain. I decided I never wanted to spend another Thanksgiving morning in that manner. Fortunately, that calamity befell neither me nor any of my patients again, and I have never again neglected to perform the sphincterotomy.

Cutting this muscle does not, as some might suspect, cause incontinence, because it is cut at a right angle and only at one location. And we do not pack the rectum. It is the packing of the rectum with cotton, a procedure still followed in many places, that causes loss of bowel control. Packing the rectum keeps the severed muscle fibers separated so that they cannot naturally grow together again.

Many general surgeons still do not know that this muscle should be cut. That is why their patients have so much pain, postoperative narrowing of the rectal outlet, and frequent fecal impaction.

Pilonidal Sinus

The diagnosis of pilonidal sinus is not difficult, and some patients even make their own diagnosis. These cases are very easily

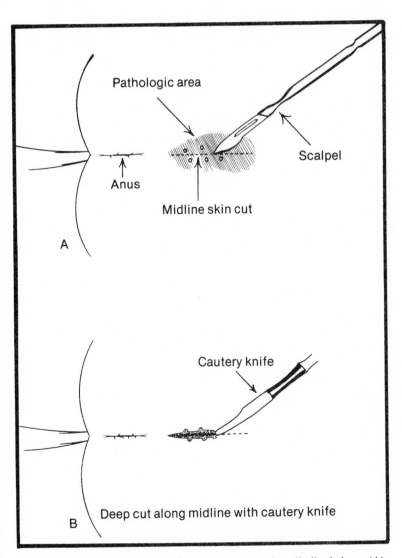

Fig. 11. The cutting performed in proper surgery for pilodinal sinus: (A) light skin incision with scalpel followed by (B) deep incision with hot knife.

taken care of in the office. Using a twenty-five-gauge five-eighth-inch needle, inject 1 or 2 cc of a local anesthetic (xylocaine or lidocaine) just beneath the skin of the sacro-coccyxgeal area to create a wheal. The anesthesia need not be deep. Usually very little anesthesia is required, on the order of 5 cc to 10 cc, and should be administered beneath the wheal with a twenty-gauge one-inch needle. Allow about three minutes for it to take effect.

Always make your incision right on the midline, as shown in figure 10. Carry it far enough anteriorly, beyond any involved tissue, and carry it far enough posteriorly. Always go deep down to the periosteum of the sacro-coccygeal bones. This incision divides the fibrous jacket of the sinus into two portions of unequal size. You now have the sinus opened like a book.

You then proceed to separate the skin from the fibrous layer. This can be done with blunt dissection. Remove no skin and as little as possible normal tissue. Be sure to remove all fibrous and pyogenic material; failure to do so will chance a possible recurrence—which happens too often. To differentiate normal from abnormal tissue is not difficult for the experienced operator. I will not say you can shell out a pilonidal sinus, but once it is raised from its bed, normal and abnormal tissue can usually be distinguished quite easily.

Do not make a wide incision, just one midline cut. The rest of the cutting is cutting beneath the skin. The length or the depth of the wound does not affect healing; however, a wide wound does heal slowly. An operation done in this manner but without a wide incision heals very rapidly, and the scar is usually only one sixteenth of an inch or less in width. If the surgery is done correctly, packing the wound is superfluous. If the patient originally appears with a pilonidal abscess, open and drain this at least three days before surgery.

After surgery keep the wound clean. Have the patient sit in hot water for ten minutes three or four times a day. If, as very rarely happens, granulation tissue appears, excise it with a scissors or curette it with a scalpel.

Diverticulosis

A diverticulum is a sac or indentation like a large pockmark occurring in the wall of the descending colon. When present, these identations can be quite numerous, and they are present in over 20 percent of all people over forty years of age. Often they present no symptoms. The cause of diverticulosis is probably congenital, like hernia, and although the tendency for diverticula to develop is present at birth, they usually do not show up until many years later. This condition is positively identified on barium X ray, but the patient's symptoms are highly suggestive: vague aches and pains in the abdomen come and go with no particular pattern. These pains probably result from concretions of fecal material trapped in these sacs and causing a low-grade infection.

Diverticulitis

When diverticula become infected, diverticulitis develops. You would think in the presence of infectious organisms this would be very common. Actually, such is not the case, as diverticulitis is not nearly as common as diverticulosis. The major symptom of diverticulitis is constipation. The danger here is that a harsh laxative can increase the pressure in the bowel and cause a "blowout" through the diverticula, thus causing peritonitis. Bowel obstruction can occur, and if this happens surgical intervention might be necessary. The patient with diverticulitis should avoid harsh laxatives. He should do all he can to keep from becoming constipated, especially avoiding those foods which he knows constipate him. He should try to move the bowels regularly, perhaps after breakfast each day. If he fails to have a bowel movement, an enema is in order, a low enema given while sitting on the toilet.

If obstruction threatens, a liquid diet should be chosen. A high-residue diet must be avoided (seeds and roughage such as celery, apples, cereal, and cabbage should be avoided, as should condiments). This condition is with one for life, and, though not fatal, it can only be controlled and not cured. Patients with this condition will find that to relieve gas a preparation such as Donnatal or any other smooth muscle relaxer will help.

Sigmoidoscopy

I do not routinely perform a sigmoidoscopy on every patient who walks into my clinic, nor do I order barium enemas and extensive X rays on all these people. Once again I can hear the hospital doctors wailing and hollering.

People with rectal problems and rectal symptoms are fearful. Many are in great pain, and they do not want to be unnecessarily probed, pushed, and hurt. Naturally, if my history and physical examination causes me to be even slightly suspicious of a malignancy, these tests are immediately performed. Perhaps 10 percent of my rectal patients undergo a sigmoidoscopy, a barium enema, and X rays. But if no such suspicion exists, I simply treat the condition at hand. If all the symptoms do not clear up in three weeks, further tests are ordered.

To my knowledge I have not missed a single case of carcinoma. Twice in over 3,000 rectal cases I have been three weeks late in making the diagnosis of cancer, but I do not feel that the length of these two people's lives was shortened one day by my three-week delay in making the diagnosis. I do know, however, that 2,998 patients were spared the ordeal of a sigmoidoscopy and the expense, loss of time, and great discomfort of barium enemas and X-ray examinations.

An old medical adage advises, "Doctor, if you cannot do your patient any good, at least do not do him any harm." I think 2,998 unnecessary procedures would have done a lot of people harm. But do not misunderstand me: these tests should be performed if they really are indicated.

IX

Hernia—For Doctors

At the risk of bringing down upon my head the resentment and hatred of the entire medical community, I am going to go into a detailed explanation of the technique and method of the non-surgical treatment of rupture that has been performed by a handful of men for 140 years. Doctors who have professional reputations to maintain should study the facts presented here before they sound off against injection treatment.

Surgical failures are far too frequent, pain and suffering too great, and time lost from gainful employment too long to permit thoughtless criticism of a treatment that can eliminate these hazards in most cases of hernia. The successful injection of a hernia undoubtedly requires more skill and more dedication than does the operation: it is no field for the amateur. Yet a good many doctors have attempted to treat hernia by the injection method without having sought instruction in the technique. It is the bungling of these amateurs that accounts for the condemnation of ambulatory treatment by many doctors who have never seen a skilled surgeon perform the treatment. I say surgeon—of course it is surgery. There is not a word about cutting, dissection, shedding blood, or stitching in Webster's definition of surgery.

Doctors who say the injection patient will have to undergo surgery eventually anyway should spend a week in my clinic. Perhaps then they would say, as I do, that many victims of hospital surgery will have to undergo injection treatment eventually anyway. And the scar tissue caused by the previous surgery makes my work on these poor souls far more difficult.

In 1948 Leigh F. Watson, M.D., Fellow of the International College of Surgeons, published a book covering all aspects of hernia. He included in it over ninety pages on the treatment of hernia by the injection method.

In 1954 I accepted an invitation to visit Dr. Watson in Los Angeles, where I watched him treat both men and women for hernia by the injection method. This was one of the most valuable and instructive two-week periods of my life. At that time I had been treating hernia by the injection method for four years and had about a hundred cases to my credit. I had observed three men do the work and had read everything I could find about this marvelous method of avoiding surgery and keeping people out of the hospital. But I learned much from Dr. Watson.

Dr. Watson, who was past seventy years of age at the time and who had done surgery for over forty years, was generous with his wealth of information and helpful suggestions. He impressed upon me the importance of a good truss and the fact that overtreatment is far better than undertreatment. He also stated that many surgical failures resulted from the fact that the surgeon operated on an inguinal hernia of the indirect type when the patient really had a direct inguinal hernia. Figure 12 shows the basis for distinguishing between direct and indirect hernia. The indirect type is six times more common than the direct inguinal hernia, but one cannot assume that everyone suffers from the more common type. Dr. Watson also pointed out to me that some patients have a simultaneous combination of direct and indirect hernia. He stressed that if the herniation comes directly through the abdominal wall, the needle surgeon must be sure to treat the internal and external rings, the inguinal canal, and, with special completeness, Hesselbach's triangle.

Few men have the expertise that treatment by the injection method requires, and surgeons who scoff at this method either have knowledge of its use only by comparative amateurs or, more likely, have no knowledge of it at all. Unfortunately, others listen to this uninformed or prejudiced scoffing.

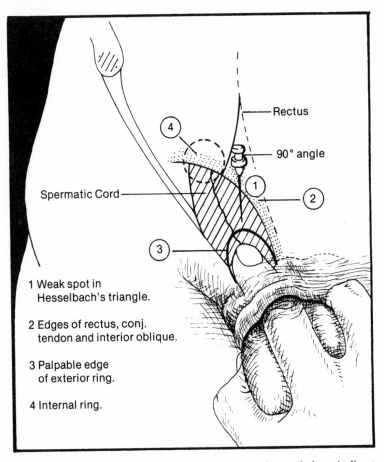

Rectus

4

90° angle

Spermatic Cord

1

2

3

1 Weak spot in
  Hesselbach's triangle.

2 Edges of rectus, conj.
  tendon and interior oblique.

3 Palpable edge
  of exterior ring.

4 Internal ring.

Fig. 12. An indirect hernia protrudes through the internal ring. A direct hernia protrudes directly through the abdominal wall at Hesselbach's triangle.

It is a sad thing, but the average general practitioner seems to look up to his surgical colleague as a godlike giver of the final word in matters of judgment on who should have what operations and treatments. He accepts all the opinions and statements of these greater men as gospel, never thinking that all hospital specialists, whether they are surgeons, anesthesiologists, pathologists, radiologists, or internists, have a vested interest in getting patients into the hospital. Thus the prejudice against the injection treatment of hernia begins with surgeons and other specialists whom the treatment would make superfluous and from them is conveyed to general practitioners who take their word for it. The public cannot decide for itself about injection treatment because doctors and the laws against medical advertising keep the public from finding out about it.

Examination

When the new hernia patient presents himself to you, first examine him in a standing position. Outline the hernia with a drawing pencil or Magic Marker on the patient's belly to determine the extend of its periphery. If possible, reduce it while the patient is standing. Note the force and direction with which the intestinal protrusion leaves the internal inguinal ring and travels down the canal, and see how much, if any, of the viscus enters the scrotum. The patient should also be examined in the supine position. Always remember that the inguinal rings and canal are farther to the side in a woman than they are in a man. Determine whether the hernia can be held in place with the examiner's middle three fingers. Boyd's Law, stated previously, stipulates that only a hernia that can be reduced with these three fingers is suitable for injection treatment. If the area covered by the hernia is so wide that it cannot be reduced with three fingers, you must refuse the case or offer the patient a limited prognosis. A hernia that cannot be reduced at all is, of course, impossible to treat.

Fitting the Truss

The fitting of the truss is most important. I rarely treat a patient unless I fit the truss myself, because treating with the wrong truss is courting failure. The doctor should not treat anyone with an elastic truss. The truss must be worn day and night throughout the treatment. Only sponge baths can be taken, since water would quickly rot the leather covering of the steel truss. The patient's spouse can help with the sponge baths. Because the fibrous tissue being built up must be protected until it has its full strength, the truss cannot be taken off while standing or sitting. Wearing a truss night and day for four months is difficult, but if attention to cleanliness is taken and proper padding, in the form of lamb's wool or chamois, is used, its presence becomes acceptable.

Often, after treatment a patient comes to like the truss so much that he refuses to discard it. I have occasionally told a patient I thought his hernia was too large for this method of treatment, only to have him insist that I treat him anyway. I have treated a few of these cases with the distinct understanding that the truss must be worn during strenuous activity even after treatment, but with most of these cases the complete discarding of the truss was eventually possible.

It is a good practice to have the patient wear the truss for one week before beginning injection treatment.

Injection Treatment

Injection treatment is always performed with the patient in the Trendelenburg position, because gravity gets the viscus well out of the injection site. Various parts of the weakened inguinal area are treated during separate visits. Begin by picking up the skin of the area to be injected with the index finger and thumb of your left hand, with your right hand inserting the needle through this elevated skin. When treating the internal inguinal ring and upper portion of the canal, always insert the needle at a forty-five-degree angle pointed toward the patient's feet. Figure 14 shows the respective sites for the injection of indirect and direct inguinal hernias. When you treat the external ring, the lower part of the inguinal canal, and Hesselbach's triangle, the needle should be nearly per-

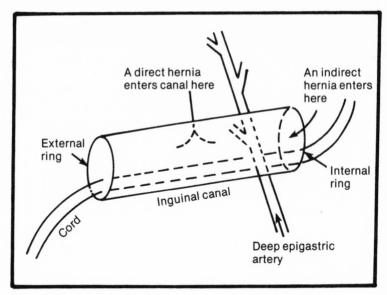

Fig. 13. An indirect hernia enters the canal through the internal ring, travels down the inguinal canal, and if complete will enter the scrotum. A direct hernia enters the canal through its posterior wall, is more rare, and will never enter the scrotum.

pendicular to the surface of the body. Never try to inject a hernia from below, through the scrotum. For most patients a twenty-gauge two-inch needle is proper, although occasionally a two-and-one-half-inch needle is used. When the needle goes through the tissues, a distinct pop is felt as it punctures the fascia of the external oblique muscle. At this point the needle should be advanced another half inch. Never fail to aspirate, because very rarely a small blood vessel can be entered. If this happens, withdraw the needle and inject the solution elsewhere. No harm has been done, because these small venules seal themselves.

A few drops of local anesthetic are usually injected prior to the injection of the fibrosing agent. This provides some anesthesia, though little, if any, is needed. More importantly, the anesthetic injection lets the physician know just what kind of tissue his needle point is in. If the fluid flows too easily, the needle is not at the

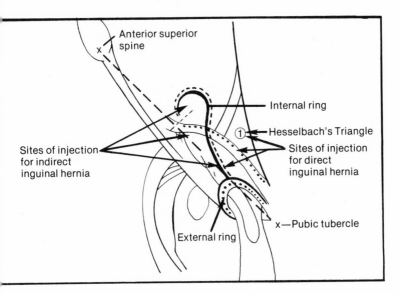

Fig. 14. Various sites for injection.

proper depth. If the resistance to the injection is too great, do not inject the fluid, because such an injection would cause pain. With years of experience the operator knows just how much resistance to his injection is correct. During the first treatment I am careful—because I know what kind of hernia my patient has, but I do not know what kind of a patient the hernia has. In other words, all people tolerate pain to different degrees. By the way, some old folks in their eighties tolerate pain better than husky fellows in their twenties. This is not a very painful experience, but naturally a needle prick in the belly is not pleasant.

At each visit following the first, the truss is removed by the surgeon after the patient has lain down; it is replaced immediately after injection. During each visit I inject the amount of solution I feel is adequate, usually from 2 cc to 4 cc. This amount will vary with the size of the hernia, its location, the speed with which the patient wants to rid himself of his truss, and the amount of complaining the patient does (a noncomplainer can be treated more quickly than one who cannot tolerate the least discomfort).

The normal length of treatment is about twenty weeks. Injections are given once weekly for twelve weeks, then every two weeks for six more weeks. The truss is worn for six weeks after the final injection. Alternative schedules are, however, possible. Injections can be given every three, or even every four, weeks—but the patient must recognize that this will prolong the wearing of the truss.

A third type of schedule can be used for patients whose stoic disposition eliminates the obstacle that soreness in the belly usually presents to more frequent insertion of the needle. This schedule is of special value when the patient lives a considerable distance from the doctor. A multiple injection method has been developed which allows two or three injections to be given through one skin puncture during each treatment: the needle is left in place while the syringe is disengaged and refilled for another injection. Treatments can be given every third day, enabling patients who live far away to receive four multiple injections during a ten-day stay near the doctor and then return after three weeks for another ten days and four more multiple injections. The patient may then return home, where he continues to wear the truss for six weeks.

But no matter what treatment schedule is used, the number of injections necessary will depend on the case. It might take ten injections or it might take twenty. The course of treatment is completed when all weak portions of the inguinal rings and inguinal canal have been closed. Palpation with his fingers gives the doctor a good idea of the amount of fibrosis that has been produced. With the patient standing, the doctor carefully feels with his fingertips the entire region of the hernia, and if a little of the sac remains it can be felt as a small, bulging, soft spot that pops in and out when pressed with the finger. Patients should be warned not to cough or strain to test this area until the injections are completed and there is a broad firm area of induration around the rings and the inguinal canal.

The Truss

A steel hood truss is used throughout treatment; a variety of sizes of trusses and a variety of sizes and types of pads should always be kept in supply. The body tries to repair itself, and on occasion a small hernia can be repaired if a good truss is worn tightly for a year or so. Never allow the patient to tell you what kind of a truss is going to be worn or when it is going to be worn. If you do this you and your patient will both be unhappy. I find that patients are very cooperative in this regard and I generally get along very well with them. Furthermore, I find that if you do a good job they will send their friends to you.

The Solution

An ideal solution for the injection treatment should be (1) practically painless, (2) nontoxic to the patient, and (3) capable of promptly proliferating fibrous nonabsorbable tissue. Years ago, when there were thirty or forty men doing this work in the United States, several drug companies made good fibrogenic solutions. As demand for the product diminished, these companies stopped making this type of medicine. I have had to use my knowledge of chemistry to recompose the solution for my own use.

How does the injection of such a solution cure a hernia? The cure for hernia is accomplished by tightening the hernial rings, closing the inguinal canal snugly over the spermatic cord, and disposing of the sac. The injection produces a general fibrosis which unites the external oblique muscle, the internal oblique muscle, and the transversalis muscles and fascia. Thus the sac is obliterated, and only a narrow pathway remains for the passage of the spermatic cord. This result can be obtained equally well by a hospital surgical operation or by means of the injection method.

The Advantage of the Injection Treatment
of Hernia in Older People

Obtaining good results when treating older people provides some of the great satisfaction that comes from doing this work. These people seem to tolerate trusses very well, and in my experience fibrotic tissue builds more quickly in older people than in the young. Their metabolisms are slower, and their systems are not as likely to pick up and carry away the fibrosing solution before it has a chance to build up fibrous tissue. Overtreatment is better than undertreatment because the amount of fibrous tissue formed by each injection varies and no harm occurs from giving one or two extra treatments. I like to tell people, "You can break one stick over your knee, and maybe you can break two sticks over your knee, but it is almost impossible to break fifteen sticks over your knee." That is the way it is with treating a hernia—the more tissue built up the better, and older people seem to build it up more easily.

A recent surgical textbook gives these death rates for men after the hospital repair of inguinal hernia:

70-79 years	1.6%
80 and over	3.3%

Thus the average death rate for men over seventy undergoing hospital surgery for hernia repair was almost 2.5 percent or one man out of forty. But I have never known of a death brought on by injection treatment.

Femoral and Umbilical Hernias

Femoral and umbilical hernias can also be treated by injection. Naturally, a different type of truss must be used, although it is worn for the same length of time.

At first visit the patient is asked to stand. The surgeon's fingertips should push the hernial contents in and out to determine the direction and force of the protrusion. As in the examination for

94

inguinal hernia, the surgeon reduces the hernia with the patient both standing and supine; and while the examining finger is in the hernial ring, he traces the ring outline on the skin with a Magic Marker. Outlining the hernia in this way helps to locate any additional weak spots in the Linea Alba; it also enables the physician to determine the circumference of the hernial sac. Then an umbilical truss must be fitted and worn at all times, except when the patient is flat on his back on the surgeon's table.

Usually, anesthesia is not needed during treatment, but a little ethyl chloride sprayed on the skin will make it numb. A small needle is inserted at a forty-five-degree angle. With the tip of the index finger in the hernial ring, the needle is guided into the firm fascia of the umbilical ring. Then very slowly 1 cc of the solution is injected. Since patients tolerate pain well in this area, if the physician uses discretion, the pain will never be severe enough to require pain pills. Once again, I like to treat the patient once a week, but occasionally I treat one twice a week or once every two weeks or even once every three weeks.

The treatment is completed when the umbilical ring is closed, the sac is obliterated, and there is no impulse when the patient coughs. Most femoral or umbilical hernias can be closed in eight to twelve treatments.

X

Prostate

There is probably no part of the male anatomy that older men have more curiosity about than the prostate gland. They assign to it powers and functions that are actually carried out by other parts of the body. Although the contrary is widely believed, the prostate gland has no real importance in sexual desire or sexual interest.

In youth the prostate gland is quite small, measuring about one and one-quarter inches by one and one-half inches. It is a solid musculoglandular body that lies immediately below the urinary bladder. The gland completely surrounds the urethra, which is the tube that carries urine from the bladder through the penis out into the world. Hard as this may be to believe, its function is not definitely known. Its secretion is concerned in some way with the vitality of the sperm. Thus its function probably is very important, for without it the conceiving of children might be impossible.

During sexual intercourse the semen comes partly from the prostate gland. Other organs that contribute to the ejaculation are the testicles, the epididymus, the vas deferens, and the seminal vesicles. So the prostate does have a sexual function, but little or no importance as a source of sexual desire.

Cancer of the Prostate

The prostate gland is a very common site for cancer in older men. It has been said that if man lived long enough and did not die from something else he would eventually die of cancer of the prostate, a statement which is made because autopsy findings in older men who died of other diseases often show the beginnings of cancer of the prostate gland. The cause of cancer of the prostate is in some dispute, but a man's sex life is not thought to be in any way a cause. Priests get it, and the worst old rounders and most promiscuous men who ever lived often do not. It is known that administering female sex hormones to old men with cancer of the gland markedly slows the cancer's growth; often these men live fifteen to twenty years with this condition, avoid surgery, and die of some unrelated condition. Cancer of the prostate almost always starts in the part of the gland toward the rectum. Therefore, it can be detected early if the doctor does a good examination through the rectum with a well-trained finger. To have a well-trained finger he must do these examinations regularly and use his brain while he is feeling. A cancerous prostate usually feels like a hard, irregular, fixed, and enlarged gland.

The diagnosis may also be made through a cystoscope, a large instrument placed through the penis and through the urinary passageway to allow direct visualization. The cystoscope examination is rarely any help, however, because by the time nodules can be seen the diagnosis can also be made quite easily with a digital rectal examination. Laboratory tests used to confirm carcinoma of the prostate, such as the serum acid phosphatase and serum alkaline phosphatase tests, show normal results unless bone metastasis has already taken place. Since this indicates that the cancer has spread to the bone, most responsible surgeons will refuse to take out the prostate gland when these tests are positive, *i.e.*, elevated. In other words, since these tests only indicate that it it is too late, they are of little practical value, at least as far as the prostate is concerned.

A simple blood test that detects prostatic cancer may eventually be used routinely as a screening tool against the world's third leading cause of death for men over the age of fifty-five. A research team at Roswell Park Memorial Institute has used immunological techniques to isolate and measure acid phosphohydrolase, an en-

97

zyme secreted into the blood by an abnormal prostate gland. The test only requires a tenth of a drop of blood and is effective at detecting one-half of early prostatic cancers and 80 percent of more advanced prostatic cancers. When this test is perfected, early detection will make cures more frequent.

The treatment of choice for prostatic cancer is not radical surgery. It is impossible to remove all of the malignant gland by radical surgery, and this cutting destroys the prostatic capsule, an adherent membrane surrounding the prostate as the skin surrounds an orange. When this natural barrier is destroyed, the cancer spreads faster. Today, most urologists feel that conservative treatment is best. If there are obstructive symptoms not relieved by female hormones, a cutting operation through the urethra with the use of a cystoscope will relieve the obstruction without destroying the natural defense provided by the capsule. This operation is called a transurethral resection.

In 1895 Dr. J. W. White made the discovery that castrating men with prostatic cancer or benign prostatic hypertrophy caused both of these conditions to practically disappear. This treatment was quite drastic, but it did show that the male hormone testosterone, in too large a supply, was the culprit in many cases.

Carcinoma of the prostate has the highest incidence of any cancer in men and is the second leading cause of death from cancer in men in the United States. Nonetheless, it is not the most common ailment of the prostate. The most common ailment involving the prostate gland is simple excessive enlargement, or as we doctors know it, benign prostatic hypertrophy.

Benign Prostatic Hypertrophy

Prostatic enlargement is rare in the Orient and in India. It is not often seen in uncivilized nations, but probably 50 percent of men in our society past the age of sixty have some enlargement of the prostate—enough to at least cause some symptoms. The cause of prostatic enlargement is not known, although the supply of testosterone is known to be a factor in some cases. One set of myths,

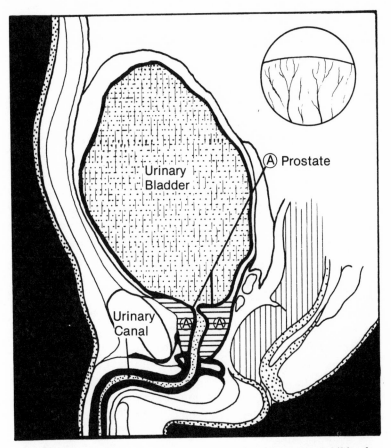

Fig. 15. Urinary bladder, enlarged because enlarged prostate inhibits the flow of urine.

of course, connects it with sexuality. But the magazine *Medical Aspects of Human Sexuality* (February 1976) has concluded that among men in their sixties there was no significant correlation between frequency of intercourse and this urological disorder.

The first symptom of prostatic enlargement is a slowing of the urinary stream. The urinary bladder loses its ability to empty itself because of the obstruction created by the enlarged gland. The residual urine increases, causing the usable capacity (in terms of being able to be filled and emptied) of the bladder to be reduced, and urinary frequency (the urge to urinate frequently) results. Figure 15 shows the urinary bladder enlarged as a result of prostatic hypertrophy. With this frequency, waking to urinate at night begins, and in a bad case waking at night to urinate can occur six or more times. Because the bladder never empties completely, a stagnant pool of urine develops, just as water that cannot drain creates a swamp in the woods. This stagnant pool is an excellent breeding ground for infection, and with this infection comes burning on urination and an almost constant urge to urinate.

I always tell patients with these problems not to decrease their consumption of fluids, but instead to increase it in order to dilute the urinary pool in the bladder. Of course, this can only be done when the urinary flow is good; one cannot keep putting fluids in when little or nothing is coming out. If the flow is poor, a retention catheter should be inserted for about a week. After a week of the copious drinking of fluids along with appropriate medication, the patient has his catheter removed. Usually, not only will the infection have cleared up, but the prostate gland very often will be found to have decreased in size. Unfortunately, most men with the problem of residual urine cut down on their intake of fluids.

Another helpful procedure for men who have difficulty in urinating is that of lying in a bathtub full of very hot water for five minutes and then pulling out the plug. As the last of the water goes down the drain, the patient usually will be able to urinate while lying on his back in the tub.

Theories of Prostatic Enlargement

1. The infection theory. There is evidence that organic infection may account for enlargement of the prostate. It is well recognized that chronic prostatitis follows in approximately half of all cases of acute gonorrhea in the male. Prostatitis can also follow acute infections occurring in other parts of the body, such as the lungs, teeth, tonsils, and kidneys. Ninety-five percent of all hypertrophied prostate tissue removed during surgery shows evidence of chronic

inflammation. I feel that poor venous return from the gland, which I will discuss more specifically later, is the chief factor in lowering the prostate gland's resistance to infection. "The rule of the artery is supreme."

2. The endocrine, or hormonal, theory. As long ago as 1895 it was known that castration, or removal of the testicles, would result in the shrinking of the hypertrophied gland and would also extend the life of any man afflicted with cancer of the prostate. As previously mentioned, this suggests that an oversupply of testosterone, the male sex hormone, is responsible for problems in the prostate gland.

3. The arteriosclerotic and varicose vein theory. With arteriosclerosis, or hardening of the arteries, there is a decrease in the caliber or gauge of the blood vessels to the prostate gland, which, receiving a deficient supply of blood, is thus not properly nourished. If varicose veins are present, venous stasis may be combined with deficient nourishment to bring on enlargement of the prostate.

Varicose veins of the urinary bladder are often noted in association with prostatic hypertrophy. These veins drain blood from the vesicoprostatic venous plexus. Bleeding from the prostatic capsule following prostatectomy is most often from enlarged veins. In the area of the prostatic capsule, a tight cover with a sphincter at each end, lymph and venous blood have difficulty circulating even under normal conditions. If the physiology is disturbed in any way, we should expect the development of venous and lymph stasis.

Some hemorrhoids are caused by varicose veins of the hemorrhoidal plexus. Likewise, prostatic hypertrophy may be due to varicose veins of the bladder, prostate, and rectum.

Other causes of prostatic venous stasis may be constipation and the consequent straining to move one's bowels, a prolonged upright position, lifting, habits which do not permit the frequent enough emptying of the bladder, and nervous tension (which produces bladder spasm, rectal spasm, and the retention of gas in the rectum). All of these conditions interfere with the proper venous return from the prostate gland.

Decompression

Once a prostate gland interferes with the flow or urine, decompression of some sort must be sought. Short of surgery, the following mechanical means are at our disposal:

1. Bed rest, which takes weight off of the gland, making both the circulation of blood around and through the prostate gland and the drainage of urine from the bladder easier.

2. The placing of a retention catheter through the penis and into the urinary bladder to allow for automatic voiding with no strain. The elimination of the residual urine pool guards against the infection of the prostate. This is usually done as a temporary measure to prepare the patient for surgery, but I feel that the relief offered in this way may, more often than surgeons expect, extend itself to constitute a major improvement, one that can make surgery unnecessary. Later I will discuss the possibility of avoiding surgery by restoring normal functioning through several days of catheterization.

3. Massage, which provides a minor decompression. The problem here is that only about 20 percent of the surface of the gland can be massaged through the rectal wall with the doctor's fingers, leaving 80 percent of the gland without benefit of even this minor decompression.

Injection Treatment

A much fuller and long lasting decompression can be accomplished by needle surgery, that is, the injection of a sclerosing agent of a mild nature directly into the gland itself. The sclerosing agent causes an infiltration of fibrous tissue which contracts the prostate gland and forces out stagnant pools of lymph and serum. The prostate, reduced in size, no longer blocks the prostatic portion of the urethra.

The injection is a very simple procedure. Following the injection of 2 cc of any good local anesthetic halfway between the anus and

102

the posterior margin of the scrotum in the midline, a twenty-gauge four-and-one-half-inch needle is inserted through this anesthetised area, guided by the surgeon's left index finger, which is in the rectum. The needle is kept parallel to the finger in the rectum as it is advanced until resistance is felt when the prostatic capsule is reached. Then the needle is advanced another three-fourths of an inch. If a pain develops in the penis, the needle tip is in the prostatic urethra and should be moved. Treatments are given at four- or five-day intervals, and a different lobe of the gland is treated during each visit. There is some swelling of the gland during each treatment; occasionally this will be great enough to require catheterization. In over 50 percent of cases, six treatments of this type give a satisfactory result. The criteria of success are: relief of symptoms, *i.e.,* burning and painful urination, frequency of urination, and retention of urine; reduction in the force needed to empty the bladder; increase in the thickness and force of the urinary stream; reduction of the residual urine to two ounces or less.

The result of the injections is not a fibrosed and hard prostate adherent to its capsule, as one might expect; instead, curiously enough, the tissue is softer than normal and can be shelled out easily if for any reason subsequent operation is ever required. If anything, the injected prostate is easier to operate on than one that has never been injected. The injection presumably produces a liquifaction of prostatic tissue, which is absorbed by the body.

An article written in the *British Journal of Surgery* (May 1966) on this method of treatment concluded the following:

1. Seventy-eight percent of the patients in their series of injection treatments were relieved of obstruction, whereas only 74 percent of those operated on were relieved.

2. There was no mortality among their injection patients versus 6.41 percent mortality in the surgical group.

3. The treatment can be given on an outpatient basis to men of advanced age who are unfit for surgery.

4. This treatment, given in the office, can reduce the case load for hospitals, freeing beds for truly sick people.

I believe that if this treatment were given a trial by experienced surgeons in all cases of enlarged prostate, it would significantly reduce the number of prostatectomies.

This method was first used by Sir James Roberts, who was surgeon to Lord Hardinge, Viceroy of India from 1909 to 1916. Lord Hardinge had a prostate problem, and Dr. Roberts reasoned that if he could inject the correct medicine into the gland a cure could be effected; apparently the method worked, for Lord Hardinge's problem disappeared. Dr. Amba Sharma of India learned the method from Dr. Roberts, and Dr. Sharma taught this method of treatment to Dr. V. D. Mathur. Dr. Mathur submitted a thesis for a master's degree on this treatment method to the University of Rajasthan, and it was accepted. My experience shows that the method has great merit, although I find it does not always do the job completely and usually a combination of treatments is necessary. These include several different kinds of pills and usually at least one intermuscular injection in the shoulder or hip during each clinic visit.

I am not saying that all prostate problems can be corrected without hospital surgery. I still refer a few people each year to the hospitals. But prostate surgery, even today, is a serious proposition. There are four different operations for the removal of the gland, none of them any picnic. One of these operations very often leaves the man sexually impotent, and the others sometimes do. All four methods can, though they do not always, leave the man incontinent for the rest of his life.

I have on several occasions had an old man walk into my clinic with a rubber catheter protruding from his penis. Twice, I recall, the catheter had been in for more than three months. These old men had been told to have their prostate out immediately, but they had refused and had finally ended up in my clinic. After four weeks of treatment, in each case, I was able to take out the catheter. Today these men are doing fine, urinating on their own, and still in possession of their prostates. I do not say that my treatment is perfect; I admit I occasionally send people to the hospital for prostate removal. But I do wish to make the important point that usually no attempt is made to give these men a chance to avoid very debilitating surgery late in their lives. I just wonder how many of the physicians doing this "hurry-up" surgery would want to be treated that way themselves.

It has always seemed strange to me, but it appears that if there is a surgical remedy for a condition, little effort is made to find non-surgical relief. Prostate surgery is common; in men past sixty-five it is one of the most common—and serious—operations. The operation, even when successful, frequently renders men impotent.

The consensus of opinion is that retropubic and suprapubic prostatectomies (in both of which the prostate is reached through an incision in the front of the body, just above the pubic bone), results in impotence in 15 to 20 percent of patients. After perineal prostatectomy, when the incision is from below—between the anus and the scrotum—30 to 40 percent of patients will be left impotent. When the gland is only partially removed through the penis—*i.e.,* transurethrally—impotence may result in only about 5 to 10 percent of patients.

The mortality figures are thought-provoking also. The following shows the surgical mortality rate by age groups for the various operations:

	Under 60	60-69	70-79	Over 80
Suprapubic prostatectomy	0%	12.5%	13.2%	20.0%
Retropubic prostatectomy	0%	5.8%	9.0%	14.2%
Perineal prostatectomy	0%	2.3%	3.0%	4.1%
Transurethral prostatectomy	.4%	2.2%	2.3%	5.0%

As one can see from this table, surgery on older people is hazardous and should be avoided in all but the most compelling circumstances.

Prostatic enlargement does fluctuate; this is, a man may have great difficulty urinating one day and a week later urinate with considerable ease. A physician examining such a patient with a cystoscope or even through the rectum, with his finger, will find a noticeable change in the size of the gland. It often happens that in the hospital a surgeon inserts a catheter before surgery on the prostate, and after several days' use of an indwelling catheter, the patient urinates very well with the catheter removed. Unfortunately, the surgeon then goes ahead with the operation. It is my contention, and I shall call this Boyd's Rule, that if the patient is sent home at this time and if his blood urea nitrogen (BUN) and his nonprotein nitrogen (NPN) are checked monthly with no further evidence of obstruction, he is not a candidate for surgery.

Today we have at our disposal medicines that eradicate most urinary infections. We have drugs that can decongest, or, in other words, lessen the water content and inflammation of many parts of the body, including the prostate. I maintain that far too little effort has been expended in this direction, and we as physicians owe to our patients some non-surgical direction in our efforts. For too long, thinking has been surgical, and nothing but surgical. I have seen too many men come into my clinic with tears in their eyes because complications from prostate surgery had condemned them to wearing a diaper for the rest of their days. Others appear with a complaint of loss of sexual ability following this surgery. I am forced to say to these poor souls, "Sorry, I cannot help you." Any surgeon or physician of any type who questions the above should spend a week with me.

Chemical Treatment

In 1972 a report came out of Stanford University, in Palo Alto, California, on a new medical treatment for prostatic enlargement. Dr. William R. Fair, in the surgical department of that distinguished university, reported that medrogestone, a chemical homologue of the female sex hormone progesterone, looked as if it could be the drug of choice for the nonsurgical management of prostatic hypertrophy. This medicine can be given by injection in the arm or taken orally. From 1972 through 1975 I have called Dr. Fair in California several times, trying to get a supply of medrogestone. The answer has always been, "Sorry, doctor, the Federal Food and Drug Administration will not release it." I am forced to use a substitute which occasionally has some minor side effects that medrogestone is free of. This is a typical example of bureaucratic meddling. Tests are done for many years at great expense, while poor sufferers are forced to go through surgery and, yes, even die because someone or some group, probably with a vested interest, blocks still another potential nonsurgical treatment method.

Still another nonsurgical treatment that is far past the experimental stage is that developed at Rutgers University's prestigious Waksman Institute. Dr. Carl Schaffner, of the Rutgers University staff, states that candicidin, a drug that lowers cholesterol levels in the human body, shows great promise in the treatment of benign prostatic hypertrophy. It is well known that some prostatic enlargement is caused by excessive levels of cholesterol.

Candicidin was first tested on human beings with prostate disorders in England by Dr. Ian Sutherland Jones in 1968. With sixty-five patients, his success rate was 70 percent. That year Dr. Lazarus Orkin, a New York urologist, used the drug on forty-three patients, with an 89 percent success rate.

In 1972 Dr. Jesse Keshin, also a New York urologist, tested candicidin on 92 patients, 73 percent of whom improved enough to avoid surgery. In January 1975 Dr. Andrew Sporer, of the New Jersey College of Medicine, concluded a study on 100 patients treated with candicidin. He stated that 70 percent improved so much that there was no need for surgery. Since there are about 12 million men in the United States having a significant prostate problem, a method of treatment with no bad side effects which might cure 70 to 90 percent of these men would be a great boon.

The surgery and hospital bill for a prostate operation runs at least $1,500 and often over $2,000. The patient must be away from his employment for eight to ten weeks. Add to this the possibility of death and the shock to the body's well-being from which many patients never completely recover, and you have a problem that begs for a solution. It is my opinion, based on thirty years of medical experience, that the federal bureaucrats will not allow this drug, candicidin, like medrogestone, to be released for general use by general practitioners on their poor elderly male patients.

Dr. Igor Tereshin, of the Soviet Union, director of Leningrad's Research Institute of Antibiotics, began using candicidin with good results on prostatic hypertrophy cases after visiting Dr. Schaffner in 1969 at Rutgers. In conversations I have had with Dr. Schaffner, he has stated that you can get the drug in many parts of the world but you cannot obtain it in the United States, where it was developed and its efficacy was proven. Dr. Schaffner also told me that a physician who is probably the best-known cardiac surgeon in New York City (and the man who, incidentally removed my father-in-law's cancerous lung in 1950) had a prostate operation in early 1975 through the penis—that is, a transurethral resection. This surgeon feels that his problem is coming back, and so he is himself taking candicidin now—because he wants no part of further surgery. So the big shots can get the drug, will get it, and will use it on themselves. Meanwhile John Q. Public, the little man, will have to continue to submit to surgery that in many, if not most, cases could be eliminated. Such is the fate of the little man, the forgotten man in our American society.

Cryosurgery

Another method of treating urinary obstruction caused by prostatic enlargement is not strictly nonsurgical, but requires the use of special sophisticated equipment. Liquid nitrogen at a temperature of lower than 250 degrees below zero is used to freeze the prostatic tissue and destroy that portion nearest the urethra, thus relieving its pressure and allowing the urine to flow. A metal probe containing a compartment for the liquid nitrogen is introduced through the penis. The surgeon can tell where the insulated portion of the probe is by a nipple on the probe, which he can feel when his finger is placed in the rectum. The probe is insulated except for one and a half inches at its tip. This is the part that must be kept in contact with the prostatic portion of the urethra. Once the probe is in the proper position the nurse turns on

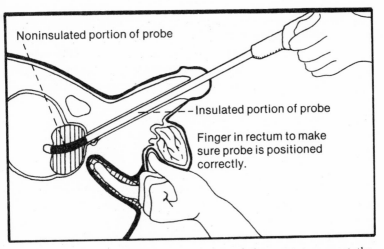

Noninsulated portion of probe

– Insulated portion of probe

Finger in rectum to make sure probe is positioned correctly.

Fig. 16. Cryosurgery to freeze the portion of the prostate nearest the urethra and relieve pressure on the urinary stream without surgery. The noninsulated (black) portion of the probe contains liquid nitrogen at a temperature below –250°C.

the liquid nitrogen. I find that a three-minute freeze is long enough. After superficial thawing, accomplished by turning off the nitrogen and turning on a heating wire, which also runs through the probe, the probe may be disengaged from the frozen portion of the prostate and withdrawn. Figure 16 illustrates the use of this probe in cryosurgery.

The objection patients have to this method of treatment is that a catheter must be left in place for at least five days after treatment. This is necessary because swelling occurs for several days after treatment, until the tissue destruction has been accomplished. The clearing of the passageway is accomplished probably through liquefaction and hemorrhagic necrosis. This method of removing offensive prostatic tissue was mentioned in a *Reader's Digest* article in December 1971.

Another benefit of cryosurgery has been explored by Dr. Rubin H. Flock, M.D., professor and head of the Department of Urology at the University of Iowa College of Medicine. Dr. Flock found that not only could he freeze and destroy the primary prostatic carcinoma mass with the cryosurgical probe, but that strangely enough the spread of the cancer was slowed much more after this treatment than similar cases treated with radical surgical. Thus some strong evidence exists that when prostatic tissue is frozen an immunological reaction takes place that has a deterrent effect on metastasis.

Despite the amply proven value of cryosurgery, in June of 1973 I had to hire a lawyer and have patients go with my attorney to the state capital in Harrisburg, Pennsylvania, to testify to the efficacy of this method of treatment. The hearing officer finally found in my favor and now Blue Shield in Pennsylvania pays $250 for this method of treatment. The following is a newspaper account of this verdict, from the York, Pennsylvania, *Daily Record* (June 25, 1973), calling it a "breakthrough." It is no fun and not cheap to constantly fight the Establishment. But what other choice do I have? A lawyer friend of mine said to me once, "Doctor, why don't you get in step with the other doctors?" My reply was, "Sorry, Horace, but down inside of me, somewhere I hear a different drummer."

JUNE 25, 1973—Loganville's Dr. Nathaniel W. Boyd scored "something of a breakthrough" when an initial determination by Pennsylvania Blue Shield denying coverage of treatment by Dr. Boyd was reversed, and the carrier instructed to adjust its payment to the patient under the Medicare program.

Blue Shield, the Medicare carrier, had based its denial on the position that the method of prostate cryosurgery used by Dr. Boyd was not a generally accepted form of treatment. But the Medicare hearing officer, C. Arthur Tress, had determined that the procedure is an acceptable one under the Medicare program and is eligible for Medicare coverage.

Atty. John W. Thompson Jr., who represented the doctor and his patient at the Medicare hearing, explained that, heretofore, Blue Shield had summarily dismissed claims for treatment not directly listed in its schedule of fees as being "not generally accepted procedure."

The hearing officer determined the procedure is acceptable and, further, that "Dr. Boyd's charge of $250 had been within the prevailing charge range in the locality for similar surgery and had not been higher than the amount the carrier would have paid to its own policyholders and subscribers for a comparable service under comparable circumstances.''

Prostatitis

The term *prostatitis* has been used over the years to label a wide variety of symptoms thought to be due to the prostate gland. I have seen men in their thirties on medical disability from the armed services who were collecting and presumably would continue to collect a hundred or more dollars a month for the rest of their lives because of so-called service-connected chronic prostatitis. I think most of these men are malingerers and are taking Uncle Sam for a ride. The diagnosis is difficult to disprove, but I fail to see how prostatitis could affect so many young men so seriously. Prostatitis is a garbage-can diagnosis, a catchall for use when the doctor does not know what else to do with a complaining patient.

Acute bacterial prostatitis is characterized by sudden onset of chills and fever, low back pain, pain between the scrotum and the anus, and painful urination. The doctor examining a prostate so afflicted will find it tender and swollen and usually warm.

The treatment of this condition can be accomplished in ten days of sulfa-drug therapy with the forcing of fluids. For chronic bacterial prostatitis, a new drug, trimethoprim, seems to be effective. This agent seems to be better than the older sulfa drugs in crossing the prostatic capsule barrier, which to some extent blocked the effectiveness of previous medicines. Thus for the first time a medication is available that can offer a cure for chronic bacterial infections of the prostate gland. Perhaps this progress in the chemical treatment of prostatitis will encourage new interest in other medicines for the prostate, together with the release to physicians of those drugs already proven successful against other prostate ailments.

XI

Other Conditions Helped By Nonsurgical Treatment

Varicose Veins

Varicose veins are veins that have become permanently dilated and whose valves have been destroyed, rendering them unable to support the column of blood and to perform their proper function, that of transporting blood back to the heart. As a rule, the disease is confined to one or more segments of the vein, which are dilated and increased in length, so that they become convoluted; all the coats of the vein are thickened, chiefly by an increase of connective tissue.

Although many varicose vein patients have no symptoms to complain of, the likely symptoms include heaviness, fatigue, itching, tingling, numbness, and sometimes cramps in the extremities. Dermatitis is most marked just above the internal malleoli, or anklebone. The discomfort the patient may feel bears no proportion to the extent of the varicosity, and when the pressure is not high there is little suffering. The usual complaint is a sense of weight and fullness in the limb after standing or walking.

One of the serious effects of the vein's reduced ability to carry blood is that tissue in the area of the varicosity is poorly drained and thus becomes, in effect, poisoned by its own wastes. The tissues swell like a swollen ankle, and if things get bad enough an ulcer develops. I have seen many people with these ulcers given antibiotics, a treatment which does no good because it does not remove the cause of the ailment. What must be dealt with is the

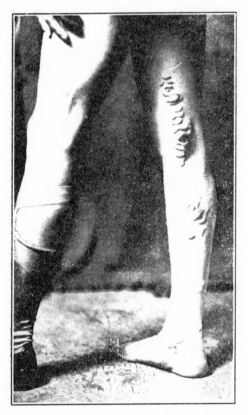

Fig. 17. Varicose veins suitable for injection treatment.

static circulation. The surgical stripping of the veins involved has much merit and is an improvement over the old saphenous ligation (or "tying-off") surgical treatment much in vogue fifty years ago. There probably will never be a perfect treatment for varicose veins. Perhaps a vein bank could be established, where veins from young automobile-accident victims could be stored for later use as replacements for severe varicose veins.

Many of the people I have seen as varicose vein patients have already had hospital surgery and are not 100 percent satisfied.

Some of these people can be helped by injection, although some will not find further improvement if this method is attempted. Nonetheless, in many cases these veins can be safely destroyed either by surgery or injection treatment, because they are doing more harm than good in their varicose condition. They can be eliminated as a source of trouble, and the deep veins still in good health can handle the entire job of supplying nutrition to the leg.

What is the cause of varicose veins? Probably our erect posture has something to do with their cause. It is generally recognized that man spent much of his time on all four limbs until the last few thousand years. Prolonged motionless standing certainly is a cause. The kneading action of the muscles of the leg against the vein wall during walking helps the valves of the veins to do their work. Pregnancy certainly helps bring on varicose veins, tight circular garters are a factor in some cases, and extreme obesity is often a cause. Heredity is a factor; several members of a family in succeeding generations often are afflicted. Congestive heart failure, pulmonary disease, and cirrhosis of the liver may cause venous stasis, thus causing varicose veins.

Infections such as thrombophlebitis, which former president Nixon suffered from, can leave varicose veins. A direct blow to the leg, like that suffered in an automobile accident, can injure the vessel wall, making the valve in the vein unable to do its work and thus result in varicosities.

If the patient wants to treat himself for varicose veins, the best advice I can give is to avoid, if you can, all the causes. Wrap the legs with a four inch elastic bandage, and as you wrap the bandage up the leg, make it overlap, toward the knee, one-half inch on each circling of the leg. Another method that helps, especially if there is ankle swelling, is lying on your back, taking off all constricting garments below the waist, and propping the feet up on the wall by the bed so that the feet are two feet higher than the shoulders.

Varicose veins were first treated by the injection method in 1851, and most of the early work was done in Europe. In 1894, at a surgical congress in Lyons, France, the injection treatment of varicose veins was discussed. In 1908 Schiassi, of Italy, suggested a combination of injection treatment and surgery. In 1911 the development of a better injection fluid gave impetus to this form of treatment, once again in Europe. The work was begun in the United States in the 1920s.

The injection treatment of varicose veins actually converts the bad vein into a fibrous band which the body eventually absorbs. If the patient has bad varicosities and symptoms such as swelling and tiredness of the legs, aching, etc., it is probably a good idea to treat them, especially if they are large enough to "bounce back" after being pressed by the surgeon's finger. Such veins are suitable for injection with a sclerosing agent at weekly intervals, while being kept wrapped with a four-inch-wide elastic bandage during the course of treatment. Some pain, redness, and hardness will follow each treatment, but these symptoms usually clear up in four or five days. Six to twelve weekly treatments usually provide a satisfying result.

Injection treatment is indicated in the following cases:

1. Varicosities so large and painful that they partially or completely disable the patient.

2. The presence of varicose ulcers, varicose eczema (due to poor nutrition of the skin in the area of varicosity), or pruritus. These call for the injection of feeder veins.

3. Varicosities associated with arthritis of the knee or ankle.

4. Spider-web, skyrocket, and hairlike types of varicosities which are practically symptom-free but which women frequently wish removed for cosmetic reasons.

I prefer to have the patient in a standing position for the injections. A tourniquet is applied, and beginning at the lowest point of the varicose veins, an injection (or multiple injections, spaced one inch apart) is given. When the needle is withdrawn, an assistant holds a pledget saturated with alcohol to the venous opening, and a square of gauze is attached to the injected area with adhesive tape. Cellophane tape is used on sensitive skin. The gauze is removed by the patient eight hours later and an epsom salt bath (one cup of salt to a bathtub of warm water) is taken, provided the patient has no ulcer or eczema. The patient sits in the bath for ten minutes and then dries his or her lower extremities by patting only—no rubbing.

I have used most of the available sclerosing solutions and find Soricin best for large veins. Soricin is nontoxic and completely obliterates the varicosities with a very small chance of recanalization thereafter. The percentage of recurrence with this agent is low. There have been very few local, and no systemic, reactions following the use of this drug. Multiple injections can be given. The average in large veins is 1 cc, and in smaller veins ½ cc or less. The injections are given once a week.

In cases of varicose ulcers, the injection of the sclerosing solution into the feeders leading to the ulcers completely scleroses the veins, and the ulcers heal.

The advantages of the injection treatment of varicose veins, ulcers, and eczema, are obvious. The length of treatment, the time of disability, and the cost are all less than they are in surgical stripping. The treatment is given to ambulatory patients who lose no time from work. Fatalities, as far as I know, are nil; the danger of embolism from a thrombus is almost negligible because the newly created fibrous tissue adheres firmly to the vessel wall, leaving nothing to float loose in the system, the column of blood in a varicose vein is in most cases static and not moving toward the heart, and the absence of infection obviates the chance that a thrombus might disintegrate.

An alternative to the injection of sclerosing solution in cases of varicose ulcer is the injection of autogenous (the patient's own) blood in the ulcer area. Ten cc of blood is drawn from a convenient vein, and starting inside a margin one-eighth to one-fourth inch from the edge of the ulcer, the surgeon inserts the needle until it passes the resistant fibrotic area into the subcutaneous tissue surrounding the ulcer, where the blood is slowly injected. It may be advisable to anesthetize the part to be injected with 1 percent novacaine solution, injected around the margin of the ulcer.

After the injection of the blood, the ulcer is painted with a 5 percent aqueous solution of gentian violet, then dried, following which a powder consisting of zinc oxide, boric acid, zinc stearate, talcum, and thymol iodide is sprayed over the ulcerous area with an atomizer. Gauze and a bandage are applied to the area, and finally a four-inch width of elastic bandage for support.

Autogenous blood treatment is indicated in postphlebitic ulcers, ulcers in which the deep veins or intercommunicating veins are involved, and varicose ulcers that will not heal even after all the feeders are injected, as well as luetic, diabetic, arteriosclerotic, and osteomyelitic ulcers.

Hydrocele

A hydrocele is an abnormal collection of fluid in the scrotum. It can be caused by infections such as gonorrhea or syphilis, but more likely it is due to a direct injury, such as a blow to that area of the body. In truth, however, about 50 percent of hydroceles are of unknown origin. This condition almost always occurs on only one side. The diagnosis is usually easy to make. There is a swelling in the scrotum that does not go away when the patient lies down; and when felt with the fingers the swelling behaves as if it were a liquid. Cancer of the testicle, which rarely occurs, occurs as a much more solid mass, one that grows at a much slower rate than a hydrocele. Once again, there is a surgical treatment for hydrocele, and the results are usually good.

If, however, one wishes to avoid surgery, the injection treatment in the doctor's office is effective in about 70 percent of cases. This treatment does cause some pain after treatment, but usually the patient loses no working time. If the cure is going to be effected, usually one to three treatments at two-week intervals are sufficient. The technique of treatment is for the doctor to place a few drops of zylocaine, a local anesthetic, at the spot on the scrotum selected for treatment. A needle is then inserted until it reaches the fluid, which is then completely evacuated. Without moving the needle, the sclerosing agent is introduced. Difficult as this may be to believe, this is an almost painless procedure. Often one treatment is enough to keep the fluid from reforming.

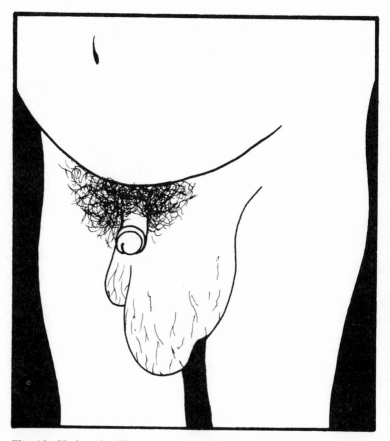

Fig. 18. Hydrocele. The scrotum is enlarged on one side, containing a great amount of fluid.

Ganglion

A ganglion is a swelling or lump located near a joint. The swelling contains a white cheeselike substance. These ganglia are usually found near the wrist, but occasionally they are found near the knee and the ankle. They are most often found in females between the ages of ten and forty.

The treatment begins by having the patient flex the wrist while a small needle is used to obtain local anesthesia. A larger needle is then introduced. The gelatinous material is then aspirated through the larger needle, and when the sac is empty, a sclerosing agent is then injected through the same needle. After the sac is fully distended, the first solution is withdrawn. Then through the same needle, a new sclerosing solution is injected and the area is sealed with a tight bandage. Some ganglion may be cured in one treatment by this method, but occasionally as many as three treatments are needed.

Bursae

Bursae are small sacs that occur normally in the human body and secrete a lubricating material known as synovial fluid. This fluid acts as a lubricant which permits the ligaments, bones, muscles, skin, and other structures to move freely. Bursae may become inflamed and distended with fluid, often as a result of injury. By reason of its location, the kneecap, or patella, bursa is the most frequently involved. Hence the name "housemaid's knee"—and prolonged kneeling can definitely be a cause. In the acute state there is swelling and tenderness over the kneecap, and the pain is made worse by flexing the knee.

The bursae over the elbow are also frequently involved. There are many other bursae in the body, but these are the most frequently affected and lend themselves best to office injection treatment, with which there is no scar and little pain. Again, a trip to the hospital can be avoided, as can all loss of time from work. The fluid is drained from the sac, and when the sac is empty the sclerosing fluid is injected.

Hypermobile Joints (Low Back)

So far every condition discussed has had a surgical remedy, albeit painful, expensive, and time-consuming. We will now discuss a condition that affects millions of people, but for which a good surgical treatment does not really exist: low back pain.

The late John F. Kennedy was afflicted with severe low back trouble originating in a naval accident during World War II. Not only was Mr. Kennedy a very wealthy individual, but as president he certainly had access to the very best surgeons and treatment available—yet no one could help him with this condition. In discussing his problem and the various forms of treatment which had failed to give him relief, he stated, "There is no such thing as a back specialist."

The number of low back sufferers are legion, and many thousands of people are affected by a restriction of motion or an excess of motion in a joint. These people can be helped by osteopathic manipulative therapy, and patients with such problems often go to chiropractors. Chiropractors are a much maligned group, and it is popular cocktail conversation to talk as if they were quacks. Well, every profession has its quacks, but I, as a person who has known many chiropractors, find that on the whole they are a very decent group who help many people who have found no relief in their dealings with the doctors of medicine. They have their failures, just as we all do. I see no reason to assume that all chiropractors are dishonest men or charlatans; on the contrary I have found that most of them are very ethical and honest. Not only that, but they are also humble, a trait I find singularly lacking in most hospital doctors—to the point that one wonders if their degree is M.D. or D.O. or if they think it is a G.O.D. degree. The manipulation given by chiropractors, like that given by old-time osteopaths, often brings relief by breaking up muscle spasms and freeing up joints that have become stiff from one cause or another.

Many back problems and hypermobile joints are, however, beyond the help that manipulation can offer. For these cases injection treatment is of great value, but to understand how and why such needle surgery works, we need to look at some aspects of the human anatomy.

The spinal column is a bony framework consisting of seven cervical vertebrae in the neck area, supported from below by twelve thoracic vertebrae, below which lie the more massive five lumbar vertebrae. (See fig. 19.) There is an opening in all twenty-four of

120

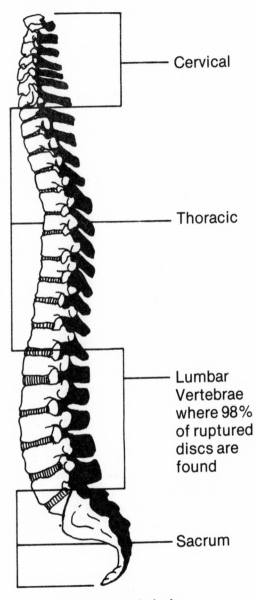

Fig. 19. The spinal column.

Cervical

Thoracic

Lumbar
Vertebrae
where 98%
of ruptured
discs are
found

Sacrum

these vertebrae, and through it the spinal cord passes. This bony armor thus protects the extremely vital spinal cord.

These vertebrae are set one upon the other with contact by facets from the vertebrae above to the vertebrae below. There are also muscles that give strength to this bony column, but the chief supporting strength comes from the ligaments that help to hold this architectural masterpiece in place. As we grow older and stop exercising—and perhaps gain a good deal of weight—this twenty-four-story building grows weaker and is less able to cope with the strains, falls, and sudden jolts it is often subjected to.

Ligamentous tissue is tough, but not very elastic. Once forcibly stretched by trauma, this ligamentous tissue is unable to snap back to its original length. This being the case, it should not be very difficult to understand how the ligaments of any joint, once over-stretched, will leave that joint in a wobbly, loose, and unstable conditon. Along with this instability very often comes chronic pain. The object of needle surgery in treating unstable joints is to inject a sclerosing agent into the ligaments, causing the contraction and thickening of the ligament, thus strengthening its supporting effect on that joint.

The treatment of hypermobile joints is based on the known fact that much pain and weakness in the low back, jaw, and knee are caused by the overstretching of the ligaments. The original research and thinking that led to a new solution of these problems by needle surgery was done by the late Dr. Earl Gedney, of Norristown, Pennsylvania, and by Dr. David Shuman, of Philadelphia, in the 1930s. Dr. Shuman is still active and in practice as an osteopathic physician. In the 1950s a medical physician named George Stuart Hackett, of Canton, Ohio, started to think along the same lines. He did quite a bit of research and wrote a fine book on this work, adding much to the findings of Drs. Shuman and Gedney. Unfortunately, Dr. Hackett is now deceased.

To treat a weak joint, the needle surgeon must be an expert in anatomy, a statement that holds true for a doctor doing any type of needle surgery. The overstretched ligaments must be located and singled out. By putting the injection directly into the offending ligament, preferably near its juncture with the bone, one can shorten and thicken it, thus stabilizing the joint. This phenomenon can be compared with the role of guy wires on a flagpole. When a flagpole is in a high wind with guy wires anchoring it to the ground, if the guy wires are loose, the flagpole is blown around. If the guy wires are tightened, the pole becomes stable. The same thing is true of a joint in the body that has become unstable due to stretched ligaments. There are some doctors who, I am sure, do not believe this can happen; but research has been done in the laboratory which confirms under the microscope that injection treatment certainly does accomplish just this.

Everyone has heard of the sacroiliac joint. Figure 20 shows the location of this famous but little-understood part of the body. Although many physicians were for a long time of the opinion that it was immovable, the doctors who first used manipulation found that it definitely did move and that often much pain in the low back resulted from its excessive motion. The injection of a sclerosing agent into the sacroiliac ligaments in four or five treatments often relieves the low back pain that has plagued a patient for years.

To treat the sacroiliac ligament, a two- or three-inch needle, depending on the girth of the patient, is inserted a half inch medial to the posterior superior iliac spine and is directed downward and slightly to the side. The site for insertion of the needle may be seen in figure 20. A distinct resistance is felt when the ligaments are reached. When no blood appears on aspiration, ½ cc of a local anesthetic may be injected, followed by ½ cc of the sclerosing solution.

Another common type of hypermobility is that found in the knee joint—the so-called trick knee of athletes. Most commonly a blow to the lateral aspect of the knee will damage the medial collateral ligament; in such cases one feels a definite insecurity when stepping down. I did a handspring for my children when I was in my early thirties, and my left knee was injured on landing. For six years, if I tapped my finger even lightly over the inside of my knee, the pain

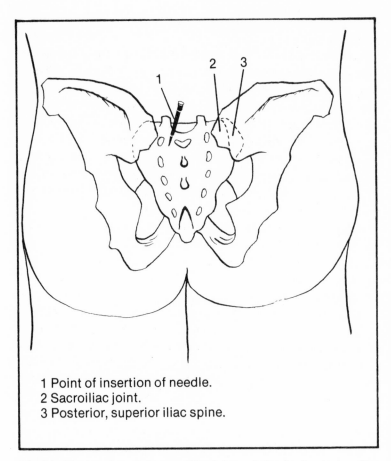

1 Point of insertion of needle.
2 Sacroiliac joint.
3 Posterior, superior iliac spine.

Fig. 20. The location of the sacroiliac joint and the site for the insertion of the needle to inject sacroiliac ligaments.

was severe, and my knee felt insecure and wobbly. I finally had this knee injected five times, and now, twenty years after the injury, I am symptom-free.

Injection may be useful in treating the type of hypermobility that results in a chronically dislocating jaw and in treating shoulder dislocations.

Ruptured Disc

Between all of the bony vertebrae described earlier are located shock absorbers composed of a material that is able to cushion most shocks the body suffers, whether the landing after an eighteen-foot pole vault, the blow to the jaw a boxer absorbs, or a fall suffered by a sixty-year-old housewife. These shock absorbers are called intervertebral discs. These discs, apportioned one between each and every pair of vertebrae from the first cervical level in the upper neck to the fifth lumbar level in the low back, contain an annulus fibrosus, a doughnut-shaped structure made up of ligamentous tissue containing in its center a semigelatinous (nonliquid) material called by physicians the nucleus pulposus. (See fig. 21.)

Some people probably are born with a tendency toward a weak annulus fibrosus. Other individuals, by a severe strain, can tear this annulus, and the nucleus will be extruded. This is called a herniated, or ruptured, disc.

The cause of back pain in a so-called ruptured disc is not pressure of the disc on nerve roots, as the orthopedic surgeons would have you believe, because the disc is absorbed by the body in a few weeks. If surgery is delayed that long, no disc will be found. It will have been digested away by the phagocytes of the body. The back hurts in such cases because once the disc has disappeared the spinal column loses vertical height and the "guy wire" ligaments become too long and loose to keep the structure stable. With instability and unwanted motion come irritation, congestion, and inflammation. The pain may stay in the involved area of the back; or if a major nerve, such as the sciatic nerve, passes through the area of inflammation and becomes irritated, pain may develop as far away as the patient's foot and toes.

Remember, the disc is gone—the bony spinal column has lost height and has thus become unstable. When a sufferer wears a corset, the symptoms abate. Of course, a corset or surgical support will not give nearly the strength of firmed and shortened ligaments such as can be produced by injection.

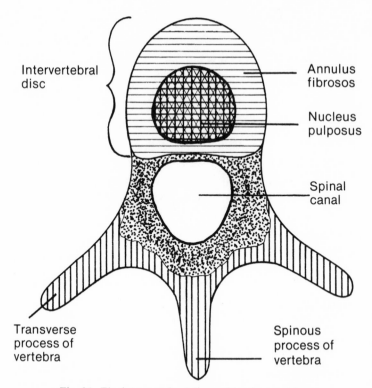

Intervertebral disc

Annulus fibrosos

Nucleus pulposus

Spinal canal

Transverse process of vertebra

Spinous process of vertebra

Fig. 21. The intervertebral disc and lumbar vertebrae.

One must not immobilize a patient with a ruptured disc. Disease begins with stasis. This is true of many maladies affecting the body, whether hardening of the arteries or the formation of gallstones. Remember, the rule of the artery is supreme. Exercise will prevent or slow down most early symptoms of disease. The better the circulation of blood in the victim of low back pain, the more quickly the phagocytes arrive and absorb the extruded nucleus pulposus; likewise, the irritation, congestion, and inflammation subside more quickly.

There are many cases on record, hundreds of cases, in which the existence of ruptured discs was proven by myelogram (a type of X ray); and though no surgery was ever performed, the patients

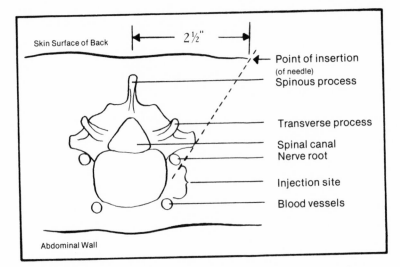

Fig. 22. The technique for the injection of a ligament in a case of a ruptured disc.

eventually recovered completely. In a certain percentage of cases, the body can repair itself. Needle surgery can speed up this process a great deal and effect some cures that the reparative ability of the body cannot.

I am not saying that a laminectomy, the surgical operation for a ruptured disc, should never be performed. The results obtained by performing this surgery can be and often are great, but results are sometimes less than good and occasionally poor. It is interesting to note that orthopedic surgeons have gotten better results since they started to do bone grafting to fuse the adjacent vertebrae after laminectomy, thus proving that even they now realize that the instability of this joint is one of the chief causes of low back pain.

When needle surgery for the disc ligament is decided upon, the surgeon should first pinpoint the involved spinal segment by using X rays. Usually a four-inch needle is sufficient. The needle is inserted two and a half inches from the midline, as shown in figure 22, and directed slowly toward the midline downward; resistance to the needle increases when the ligament has been entered, because ligamentous tissue is significantly tougher than muscle tissue. About ¼ to ½ cc of the sclerosing fluid should be injected into the ligament. Injections not placed in the ligament are of no value whatsoever.

Corticosteroid Therapy

The injection of corticosteroids for the temporary symptomatic relief of the painful inflammation of joints which is associated with rheumatoid arthritis, and in order to increase mobility in these joints, is a worthy form of treatment. The injection of these corticosteroid drugs into the joints may correctly be called needle surgery, but it is not sclerotherapy, which is used to tighten ligaments or strengthen the inguinal wall in cases of hernia. Unlike sclerotherapy by injection, the injection of corticosteroids does not alleviate mechanical damage in the body, but the suppressive effect of these substances on the process of inflammation might result in a lessening of long-term damage within the joint.

Besides being used in cases of rheumatoid arthritis, corticosteroids are also used to alleviate inflammation in cases of osteoarthritis, gout, chondrocalcinosis, shoulder tendinitis, and elbow epicondylitis. The customary dosage is about 1 ml., but less in the small joints of the hands and feet, and more (2 or 3 ml.) in the hip joint.

Chymopapain for Lumbar Disc Disease

In its twelve-year career the enzyme derived from papaya and known as chymopapain has been used by nearly a hundred orthopedic surgeons to treat over fifteen thousand patients suffering from back and leg pain. Most of these physicians were—and continue to be—enthusiastic about the drug's effects, even though a recent double blind study by the FDA indicated that chymopapain was no more effective than a placebo, thus causing the drug to be made unavailable in the United States. The chymopapain was injected by the surgeons with a four-inch needle into the area formerly occupied by the disc. This enzyme helped the phagocytes digest the remains of the ruptured disc and eliminate swelling and inflammation.

Dr. Lyman W. Smith, assistant professor of orthopedic surgery at Northwestern University Medical School, calls the FDA decision "totally irrational." He says, "How can you possibly compare 90 cases studied over a few months . . . with 15,000 done over 12 years?" By making chymopapain unavailable, he says, "we are condemning 150,000 persons yearly to unnecessary major operations."

Here is another form of nonhospital, nonsurgical treatment many physicians regard as having been proven effective but which for better or worse is being kept from patients with lumbar disc problems that will probably now require laminectomy. Supporters of chymopapain, patients and physicians alike, are asking Congress to look into the FDA's action.

XII

Iatrogenic Diseases

The term *iatrogenic,* strictly defined, refers to any physical or mental disease generated by the physician. It is frequently applied to disorders induced in the patient by suggestion or autosuggestion based on the physician's manner of examination or his diagnosis. A good example of this occurs when the physician tells a patient with a blood pressure of 110/75 that he or she suffers from low blood pressure and suggests that this condition requires treatment. This is really "manufacturing a patient," because 110/75 is very healthy blood pressure and, in the absence of symptoms, certainly requires no treatment; what useless nostrum the doctor gives such a poor soul for his supposed disease I do not know.

Even more importantly, however, the physician has thus made a person with excellent blood pressure into a blood-pressure cripple who will probably think for the rest of his life that something is wrong with him. An idea of this sort put into a patient's mind by a man as trusted as the family doctor is difficult to completely dispel.

Thus it is that many diseases that are really nothing or so minor that they require no treatment at all become reasons to go to the physician biweekly, weekly, or even daily. The public, who think of doctors as all-knowing, can interpret a nod of the head or a clearing of the throat as an affirmative suggestion that, yes, treatment is needed.

The term *iatrogenic disease* has also come to refer to any condition caused by the physician, including conditions occurring as side effects of medical or surgical endeavors. Thus diabetes mellitus caused by the doctor's using cortisone to treat a skin disease or a case of arthritis would fall into the category of iatrogenic disease. Most of us have heard of some case of iatrogenic disease resulting from surgery. X rays taken prior to a recent knee operation on Philadelphia Eagles quarterback Roman Gabriel, his fifth, revealed a suture needle deposited in the knee during previous surgery, apparently about four seasons before. Having worked its way into the muscles, the needle could not be safely removed and was left in place. If this needle has had a part in Gabriel's chronic knee problem, this case certainly qualifies as a typical example of physician negligence leading to iatrogenic disease.

Likewise, any complication from anesthesia administered during surgery, such as paralysis of the lower extremities following spinal anesthesia, would qualify as iatrogenic disease. Any surgical misadventure such as aspiration pneumonia and lung abscess from swallowing vomit into the lungs during surgery would qualify. A surgeon friend of mine died a year ago of congestive heart failure seven weeks after he had swallowed vomit into his lung following surgery for a ruptured intervertebral disc. The pneumonia caused by this foreign material in his lung was too great a strain. His heart finally just gave out.

But, unfortunately, one does not have to have an operation to get an iatrogenic disease. Just being in the hospital is enough to make many people ill. The Department of Health, Education and Welfare has reported that about 1.5 million patients each year spend an extra seven days in the hospital because of infections they pick up while there to receive treatment for some other illness. This adds up to ten million patient days with a cost of over $1 billion yearly for such infections, prime and costly examples of iatrogenic disease.

Another disease caused by doctors is the destruction of the granulocytes in the bloodstream of a patient taking amphetamines over a long period of time. These drugs are prescribed by the thousands by so-called fat doctors who specialize in taking fat off obese individuals. It is not physiologically sound to lose weight in this way, and my observations have shown me that after spending hundreds of dollars with these doctors, most patients gain weight again. How much better it is to lose weight through dieting and sensible exercise—and by refraining from gaining weight in the first place.

The practice of medicine and surgery is not easy and even the most cautious physician knows that occasionally he has done a patient some harm. His aim is to do as little harm as possible while doing something of a positive nature to help his fellow man.

Probably the most glaring example of iatrogenic disease occurred in hundreds of cases in Europe in the late 1950s. Physicians gave many women a tranquilizer, now famous, called Thalidomide, in the first trimester of pregnancy. I do not know why these women felt they needed to be tranquilized and why their doctors felt these young mothers-to-be needed to be tranquilized with drugs. But the result was that many babies were born horribly deformed—with no arms, sometimes stumps for legs, and occasionally fingers growing out of the arm at the level of the elbow. The U.S. Food and Drug Administration, with which I seldom agree about anything, made the right decision in not approving Thalidomide for use in this country, but ironically the decision was a fluke! Bureaucratic procrastination had kept the application for the drug's release sitting on an official's desk until the news of deformed babies started coming in from Europe.

But though I agree with the FDA decision on Thalidomide, I must add that I disagree strongly with the trend toward labeling vitamins as drugs and restricting their public availability. This action could lead to great damage to the health of the American people, many of whom need these vitamins as supplements to diets not sufficiently nourishing; this would be a phenomenon similar to iatrogenic disease—illness created by those responsible for guarding and improving health. Since most vitamins are known to have very low toxicity and few side effects even when taken in massive amounts, there is no justification for the FDA's restricting their sale in amounts that might be used as daily supplements to keep people in the best of health.

On the subject of iatrogenic disease I must add a few words about the many millions of unnecessary X-ray pictures taken each year.

All doctors know and will freely admit that these X rays are powerful and very destructive. Why else does the roengenologist wear a lead apron around his waist and stand behind lead barriers? X rays can cause sterility, and the low birth rate among these specialists confirms this.

It is well known that in a lifetime our bodies can absorb only so many roentgen units; as the body cannot rid itself of this radiation once it has absorbed it, these roentgen units cumulate in the body, eventually creating great danger of malignant diseases of the blood. Many cases of leukemia can be traced to the accumulation of too much radiation. And the sources of harmful radiation are increasing: wristwatches with radium dials now deliver it to us, as do our televisions, and perhaps our nuclear power plants. This increase provides all the more reason to cut down on unnecessary X-rays. Even moderate doses of radiation administered to children for tonsillitis or enlargement of the thymus gland have been known not infrequently to induce thyroid cancer that may not show up until 20 years later.

As a rule of thumb I would say that at least 50 percent of all X rays taken in this country are unnecessary. All of them, and all radiation treatments as well, are potentially harmful.

In the last twenty-five years I have known socially or had business contacts with four individuals who were stricken with forms of cancer for which X-ray therapy was decided upon. I had occasion to visit all of these four people in the last weeks of their lives, and found them all in torture, not so much from the cancer as from the horrible burns inflicted by the X-ray treatments. The skin of these poor men and women was burnt, dried up, and peeling. They were in constant pain. Three of them looked at me with tears in their eyes and told me, "I don't think all those damn X-ray treatments helped me a bit. They made hell of my last days on this earth, and I am sorry I ever let them do it." This is another case of the trouble caused by misguided medical practitioners when they seek to cure by the wrong means or without real concern and compassion for the patient.

XIII

Malpractice

It has become fashionable in the last few years to sue the doctor if treatment results are unsatisfactory or if the patient feels he has suffered some injury during treatment. Now, doctors are human beings; they are far from perfect. They deal every day with people's bodies. In no other profession or business is there such a unique relationship.

The personal satisfaction of any physician is great, especially if he performs surgery. However, if things do not turn out well or if the patient suffers grievous injury, the situation becomes impossible. Hell hath no fury like a patient who is worse after treatment than he was when he went to the doctor. You can have a house built, and it can fall down. You can, of course, sue the builder to recover the money that was wasted. A very simple thing indeed. But how can a doctor be expected to pay to take care of a permanently injured patient who, after brain damage, for example, might live on for thirty or forty years like a vegetable? Certainly there must be some compensation for the poor patient, but an award of over a million dollars is a burden that cannot be born by an individual in the medical, or in any, profession. The state or federal governments will have to come up with some remedy, or physicians will stop performing valuable life-saving procedures.

If a physician has been practicing surgery for over ten years and has never been sued, he has simply been lucky. Some of the most scrupulous operators I have ever known have been sued. All that is needed is a result less than perfect with some hint of doctor responsibility, or a patient who is litigation-minded and a lawyer who, because of no-fault automobile insurance, finds time on his hands.

I see no earthly rationale for the contingency fee system that is in vogue in the United States of America. What possible relationship is there between the damage the patient has suffered and the amount of work the lawyer performs? If this thinking were carried over to other kinds of services, why could not the automobile mechanic say, "I fixed your car, Mr. Fat Cat Attorney. Now you owe me one third of what you will make by being able to use your car to see your clients for the next six months." A lawyer should be paid for the number of hours he puts in on the case at an hourly rate that is commensurate with the brains needed to solve his client's problem.

Perhaps it is not surprising that lawyers are now getting much more out of malpractice suits than patients are. An analysis of the malpractice premium dollar in one state shows that the legal system receives fifty-five cents while the patient receives only twenty-three cents—the remainder, of course, goes to the insurance company.

What has gone wrong with the system? Have doctors become so sloppy and bad results so frequent that patients who have suffered some injury are now being compensated to the tune of $1 billion a year? Yes, $1 billion of the $104 billion spent for medical care each year is now returned to patients to compensate them for damages the hospitals and doctors inflict.

Not too many years ago a doctor could buy malpractice insurance, the premium of which would cost him roughly one week's salary—a big expense, but one he could live with. Now he can hardly get insurance at all, and if he can get it, it costs two or three months' net income. What can he do but raise his prices, thus making the cost of medical care even higher? It has been estimated that the public already pays an extra $2 to $3 per office visit because of the cost of malpractice insurance, and even greater costs are likely to be passed on to the patient when surgery is involved. (Strangely enough, the premiums a doctor pays bear no relationship to the number of operations he performs yearly or the amount of money he earns. Illogical as it is, the busy surgeon who performs

500 or more procedures a year pays no more than the practitioner who performs only 50 or 60.)

In a recent CBS TV "60 Minutes" broadcast, a Nevada obstetrician was interviewed because he had had the audacity to declare that he was "going bare," which means that he had decided to practice his specialty without any malpractice insurance. The physician had worked out with his lawyer a presumably legal device whereby all of his assets were transferred to a trust so that if he were sued by a patient, the patient could not collect anything.

As the doctor did not dispute the interviewer's suggestion that he earned $300,000 a year, we can assume that this figure is about right for his income. His great income notwithstanding, the doctor complained that his malpractice premiums had risen from $6,000 a year to $18,000 and he was not going to pay this increase even though the money would be totally deductible from his income tax with the result that after taxes he would not be out $18,000 at all but only about $9,000.

Here we have a man "earning" a huge sum of money each year. He is supposed to be a humanitarian, dedicated to the health and well-being of his patients, but in truth he has so little regard for them that he is unwilling to spend even 3 percent of his net income to assure their welfare in the case that some calamity should befall them following their surgery. We do not need men this greedy, this selfish, or this unfeeling in the medical profession.

My point is that high as malpractice insurance premiums may go, it is important that doctors pay the cost, not only for their own good but for the good of their patients. And as there has not been a great number of doctors "going bare," I assume that most doctors continue to be willing to pay what they must for such coverage.

A more serious threat to society is the very real possibility that insurance companies will stop writing malpractice insurance altogether. What will happen then? Will anyone be willing to be a doctor? Do not laugh; it could happen. What went wrong? Are doctors the victims? Or are patients the victims? Perhaps much of this modern trend toward legal suits against doctors comes from overspecialization, which results in the patient's often not even knowing the doctor who has operated on him. The warm doctor-patient relationship may be disappearing forever.

Physicians who do not know their patients sometimes fail to treat them with proper compassion and dignity. The haughty attitudes of some specialists cause them to be insensitive, for instance, to long patient waiting time in the office. Ninety-eight percent of the patients polled in a recent study said that they were generally forced to wait past their appointment times to see the doctor. Waits of one or two hours at the doctor's office, with no apology or explanation, are not uncommon. Such neglect of basic human consideration does not produce in the patient a willingness to indulge the foibles—or errors—of his doctor.

Doctors are also using more daring procedures than ever before, and because of this patients who ten years ago could not have been treated successfully are benefiting. But patients are at the same time being exposed to new risks. In such cases juries are awarding huge damages to patients when there really has been no negligence on the part of the doctor. Medical "maloccurrences" will happen. Often a procedure that can help a patient greatly can also cause harm because of factors that the doctor cannot anticipate. Famed heart-transplant man Dr. Christiaan Barnard has pointed out that unfortunately the threat of malpractice suits will make surgeons hesitate to use new surgical procedures and thus slow our progress in dealing with ailments such as heart disease.

Some malpractice claims are legitimate. Probably thousands of people are injured each year through physician negligence. These are often patients who undergo unnecessary surgery or have prescribed for them drugs which are known to have bad side effects. Some doctors, it is true, do ignore complaints that should be investigated. Half a million Americans are admitted to hospitals each year because of the bad side effects of drugs.

But in some cases the side effects of drugs are impossible to foresee. A certain hormone thirty years ago was routinely used on new mothers to dry up their breasts. Now, in the last ten years, we find cancer of the vagina in the young girls who suckled at their mothers' breasts as the breasts were being dried up. This side effect, however, could not have been anticipated and should not be considered a result of physician negligence.

What of the new oral antidiabetic drugs? Some authorities are now claiming that they cause premature heart disease. I feel no jury should find a physician guilty of negligence if at the time he chose it his course of treatment was generally considered safe and his treatment was obviously helping sick people. To protect themselves, doctors are now, quite naturally, practicing defensive medicine. That is, they are making the safest, and not necessarily the most beneficial, choices; they are ordering extra laboratory work to strengthen their position in case they should ever be sued, and so the cost of medical care rises a little more.

Is it possible to have a no-fault malpractice system? The Pennsylvania Medical Society is asking that a limit of $100,000 be made on awards, that binding arbitration be provided for, and that money be provided for the state's use in disciplining incompetent doctors. The governor of Pennsylvania would like to set up non-binding arbitration that could be appealed in court. Under this system the patient would have to put up a $2,000 bond which he would lose if the award went against him. This chance of losing $2,000 would, at least in theory, keep a patient from bringing a frivolous suit. Along with the other provisions of the governor's proposed solution, joint underwriting by all the insurance companies writing liability insurance in the state would provide medical malpractice insurance.

The legislatures of the various states have it within their power to solve the immediate dilemma, and they probably will, but I am not sure their solutions will be to everyone's satisfaction.

XIV

The Right to Die

Any human being who has lived over half a century has quite naturally watched loved ones grow old and die. Some people are fortunate to die suddenly with little or no suffering. Others go through months and sometimes years of turmoil, pain, and the desperate trauma of knowing they are dying and facing the unknown.

It is a horrible thing to watch a talented, intelligent, productive person revert to an infantile state, a state of mental and physical degradation in which, for instance, he may lose control of his bowel and bladder functions. For the body to contort and freeze into the position it once assumed in the womb is a frightening, dehumanizing, and disgusting experience that no thoughtful person would want for himself or for anyone else.

Yet apparently we have judges who, either because they lack guts or firsthand experience or because they are stupid and callous, say it is murder to allow these poor vegetables, who once were dynamic flesh and blood, to simply and quietly leave their misery. Instead, the precious little bit of life they have left must be stretched and stretched, though barely existing may be difficult and painful for them, has no rewards, and offers no possibility of recovery and a return to normal life.

What right do we have to torture and put these poor souls on display while we extend their lives in the hospital among total strangers whose job it is to tend them?

In the fall of 1975 several medical cases received wide publicity.

These patients, without the continued use of extensive, sophisticated, and very expensive medical equipment, would have died within minutes. They were literally being kept alive by machines.

In the much-publicized Karen Anne Quinlan case the expense was said to be $435 per day, or $150,000 per year. Who pays such expenses? Indirectly, everyone with surgical and hospital insurance does. But in my opinion the financial toll is far less severe than the emotional expense to those nearest the afflicted person. Unlike the patient, they are not unconscious, and they must endure the long and lingering death of a loved one.

Cases like that of Karen Anne Quinlan have made us aware of the idea of "brain death," the idea that life has formally ended when electrical activity in the brain ceases. The instrument used to monitor electrical activity in the brain is called an electroencephalograph (EEG). A Hamilton, Ontario, neurologist recently implanted EEG electrodes in a bowl of lime Jello. The jiggling of the Jello—caused by footsteps, the activity of an intravenous feeding tube leading into the vein of a nearby patient, and vibrations from a respirator in the room—indicated enough electrical activity to make some of the hospital personnel conclude, when looking at the measuring instrument, that there was brain activity at the source of the electrode contacts—in the bowl of lime Jello.

So we must be careful when judging the presence of life functions by the readings on our machines. Moreover, the presence of electrical activity in the brain is no assurance that any other part of the body will again be capable of even the slightest degree of normal functioning.

There is a feeling among the laity that where there is life there is hope. This attitude seems to presuppose that there will be a cure for all diseases in the not too distant future. Unfortunately, this is simply not true. People are born and people die; they always have and they always will. It is true that great advances have been made in the prevention of infant mortality and in the curing of childhood diseases. Two hundred years ago a small number of people lived to be eighty years of age, and now many people live well beyond that age. I predict, however, that in the next hundred years the number of people who live to be ninety will not be a majority of the population. So I cannot agree with the glowing reports we have heard about finding cures for everything and living on and on.

Our age span is very much dependent upon the genes we inherit from our parents and grandparents, and no magic process is going to extend it suddenly by twenty or thirty years. We can predict the longevity of some individuals if we have knowledge of the longevity of their ancestors.

The behavior of life in its last stages is similarly predictable. Physicians are not stupid when it comes to knowing whether a patient is going to live much longer. And when a patient is put on a life-support system, the doctors know which organ is about to go and barring the limited possibilities of organ transplant, nothing can change this fact.

I have heard it said, and the courts have ruled, that the doctor should not play God and "pull the plug." I say the doctor plays God by keeping a patient alive on a life-support system when there is no hope of recovery.

Francisco Franco, dictator of Spain for some forty-five years, fell gravely ill in October of 1975. For thirty-four days after his body became incapable of functioning by itself, a team of thirty-two doctors in one of Europe's most modern and best-equipped hospitals kept Franco "alive." After twenty-six days of this, several surgeons on the case rebelled against further life-extending measures, but these measures were of course continued. The doctors who continued to extend his life apparently did not sympathize with Franco's last recorded words, spoken seventeen days before his death: "How hard it is to die!"

XV

Medical Advertising

It has often been said that one of the things that made the United States great was the free-enterprise system. If a man, through his hard work and inventiveness, had developed a new product or a new way to solve some problem, he could, by publicizing this fact, compete with the old method, and in the give-and-take of the marketplace the public could choose the method or product they preferred.

When I was a medical student I occasionally heard, not from the lecture platform but in informal conversation with another student or at a dinner some general practitioner had come to share at the fraternity house, that there were a few men who were doing work that prevented hospitalization and surgery. Conversations of this nature were quickly curtailed if a faculty member approached.

After my graduation and internship I sought out those men all over the United States who, I had ascertained by careful research, were engaged in this work which the attitudes surrounding me at school had encouraged me to think of as almost nefarious. These physicians, whether M.D.'s or D.O.'s, were most eager to teach me their skills so that I could gain real expertise in their craft. In the early 1950s I spent much time out of my own office and in other doctors' offices, sometimes three thousand miles from my home, and at great expense at a time when my finances were low or prac-tically nonexistent. The knowledge I gained from these men made the sacrifices well worth while.

When I felt I had sufficient background, I began to do the work myself. I was so impressed with the results I was seeing with my own patients and those I had seen in the offices of my teachers that I thought it was a great pity that this work and its results were not common knowledge. When I think of all the products on the market in and out of the health field that are of questionable value, if not downright misleading and in some cases certainly fraudulent, it makes me wonder why both doctors and the public are penalized in such an arbitrary manner by having public communication of medical information forbidden because of an ethical rule forbidding physicians to advertise.

Why has advertising by professional men been frowned upon? The thinking appears to have been that unscrupulous doctors or lawyers would make ignorant people their victims. But are we to expect that the physician would be less honest than the people who sell well-known preparations for hemorrhoids? False claims by any advertister should be prosecuted; certainly the public must be protected from quackery. Truth is essential to the commercial value as well as the ethical value of advertising, much of which has as its purpose the education of the public regarding some product or service. If the product is a good one, word of mouth will help to advertise it; if it is a bad one, word of mouth will destroy it.

I firmly believe that medical advertising that is not false or misleading and informs the public of new treatment methods is a boon and benefit to all. Rules that infringe on the freedom of speech should be unconstitutional. They serve no useful purpose in a democracy, while they definitely restrict the public's freedom of choice. Any group that spends millions of dollars on advertising each year, as Blue Shield does, is acting in an un-American way when it is party to keeping a physician from informing the public of little-known or unknown methods of treatment. Not only does Blue Shield discriminate against the doctor who has developed office treatment methods, by paying his patients little or nothing for these treatments, but this institution also sits by and allows a group of medical politicians to enforce rules drawn up arbitrarily by hospital doctors to cut out competition and keep prices up.

The real motive behind this restriction of trade is not to protect the patient from the quack but to squeeze the office practitioner out of the medical scene because the office practitioner is a threat to the hospital doctor. If more people knew, for example, about needle surgery, many would choose this method of treatment, and the hospital boys would have fewer patients to work on.

Consider also that the hospitals in which these doctors work are largely, if not wholly, paid for with tax money—my tax money and yours—whereas I paid for the clinic in which I work. The hospital doctors are thus in effect publicly subsidized, making it all the more outrageous that they lay down so-called rules of ethics that prohibit the public from knowing about their competition. All hospital doctors profit from Blue Shield advertising, which solicits people to become members of the hospital-going public: Blue Shield does their advertising for them. In Pennsylvania alone Blue Shield spends millions each year on advertising.

Hospital doctors advertise in other ways. The osteopathic hospital in my area, for instance, regularly holds public forums on specific health problems. These programs, free to the public, typically feature a panel of physicians who discuss the causes and treatment of, say, arthritis. I believe that they offer "information regarding health care" as a "continuing community service," just as their publicity claims. But it is true as well that these programs teach the public about services it may purchase to the benefit of the physicians who sell them. And these programs are advertised in the local newspapers, as shown in figures 23, 24 and 25.

"Come and hear about hopeful aspects for anyone with diabetes," says one of the public forum ads. Isn't this doing just what I lost my license for—*inviting the attention of the public afflicted with specific diseases*? Of course it is. But what is wrong with this? I only object that they permit themselves to do what they deny me the right to do. When they do it, it is a public service. When I do it, it is unethical.

Medical advertising need not result, as some of its opponents claim it would, in unrestricted misinformation and chaos. If a physician made claims that were false, he would end up in legal trouble. This is the way it should be. My definition of professional

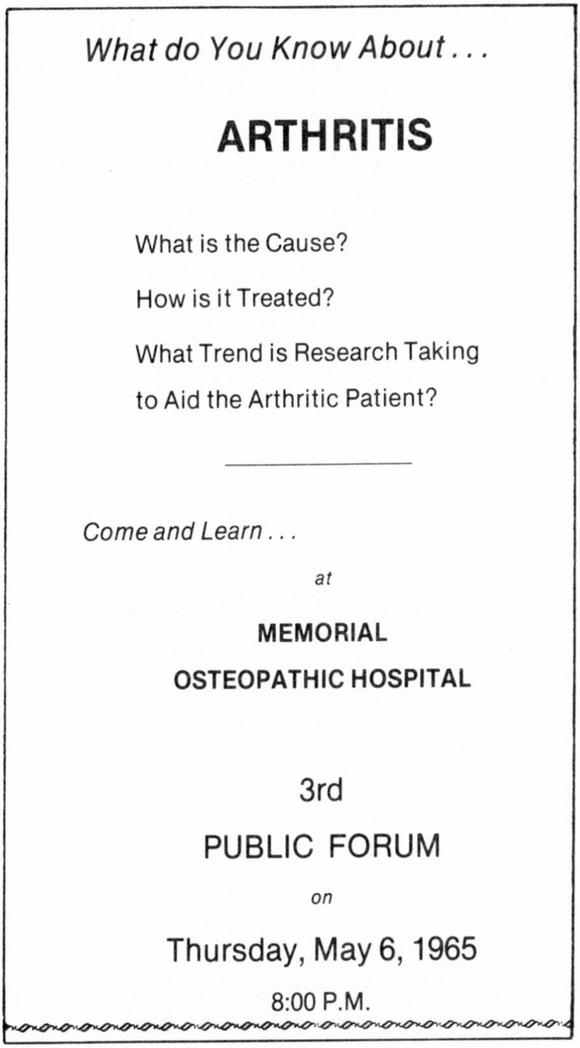

Fig. 23. Advertising that is not advertising. This "community service" makes the public aware of the readiness of both doctors and visiting nurses to help them with their arthritis—for a fee, of course. I do not say the hospital doctors should not advertise. I say if they can do it, why cannot everyone else?

CONTINUING COMMUNITY SERVICE

_____

MORE INFORMATION REGARDING HEALTH CARE

_____

MEMORIAL OSTEOPATHIC HOSPITAL

will present

The Fourth of a Series of
Free Public Forums

DIABETES

OPTIMISM and ASSISTANCE

Come and hear about hopeful aspects
for anyone with diabetes

The Visiting Nurse Association will
join us in this community service.

There will be a panel discussion,
followed by a question and answer period.

COME AND JOIN YOUR NEIGHBORS FOR THIS
INFORMATIVE PROGRAM

Time: March 19, 1964 — 8:00 P.M.

Place: Memorial Osteopathic Hospital

Fig. 24. This newspaper advertisement invites the attention of the
public afflicted with specific diseases as a "public service."

NEW METHODS

For the Treatment of

Fistula, Fissure

Hemorrhoids (Piles) and
other Diseases of the Rectum

The Gist of

Radio Health Talks

By

Dr. Frank D. Stanton
Director, The Dover Clinic

Published by
THE DOVER CLINIC
419 Boylston Street, Boston 16, Mass.

Founded in 1929 for the treatment of
Fistula and other Rectal Diseases

CLINIC OPEN DAILY
8:30 A.M. to 11 A.M.—1:30 P.M. to 3 P.M.
Excepting Sundays and Holidays

Fig. 25. Communication with the public can be for the benefit of all. Doctor Frank Stanton gave radio talks on specific diseases and invited the attention of the public to the inexpensive ambulant treatment available at his clinic. The great flow of patients this created (approximately 1,000 rectal patients per year) made it possible for the Dover Clinic to train 500 physicians in ambulant treatment between 1929 and 1958. Material from his talks was distributed in booklets which were never thought of as being "unethical."

ethics is "rules made up by those who have nothing unusual or different to offer the public, to keep those who have something unique to offer the public from letting the public know about it." If a new treatment technique is a hospital procedure, it gets press coverage by devious means—as a news story. The hospitals call in the press, for example, to tell them about heart transplants. Heart transplants pose no threat at all to established treatment methods; in fact, in the many years since the first transplants very few really have been performed. If needle surgery methods received the publicity that heart transplants receive the public would demand treatment by these methods. And so it has become not only unethical but illegal to inform the public of the existence of these methods. Recently, however, cases involving professional advertising have been appearing before the courts. Hopefully, more cases will come up, and the result will be a more sensible attitude toward advertising in the near future.

On June 23, 1975, a lawyer in New York City filed a civil antitrust suit, charging that the ban on advertising by lawyers is causing him and other lawyers to suffer substantial economic losses, because of which they face extinction unless the ban is lifted. The lawyer, Carl Person, stated he wished to advertise his hourly rates and legal specialties. He claimed that the high prices charged by well-known law firms discouraged potential clients from seeking legal aid. Mr. Person acknowledged the fact that he faced disbarment if he solicited clients under the present system.

The week that Person filed suit for the right to advertise, the United States Supreme Court ruled by a vote of 7 to 2 that it was legal for doctors to advertise abortions. What a paradox for the court to rule that it was legal to advertise one form of medical procedure only, when this one procedure had been itself illegal just four years before!

This same United States Supreme Court, comprised of the same nine men, following the lead of the Pennsylvania Supreme Court, had refused to hear my case a short time before. A lower court had ruled it was illegal for me to print a little booklet telling the public about treatment methods that didn't require people to be confined

148

in hospitals. If you do abortions, a procedure that requires no great skill, you can advertise. If you are one of the few men who know how to keep hundreds of people out of the hospital each year, you are not allowed to let the public know about it. Across the nation people are crying out for improvement in medical care. But how can we ever expect our medical care to improve if in order to preserve a good thing for the fat cats of our society, those high in the Establishment, we have resorted to methods that not only are expensive but in effect deprive many citizens of the freedom to choose a physician and a treatment method?

Rules against medical advertising, or against medical education and enlightenment, penalize many people.

1. Patients with heart trouble, high blood pressure, diabetes, etc.—whose bodies cannot stand the rigors of hospital anesthesia and surgery—are either doomed to surgical treatment or have to put up with and nurse their ailments forever.

2. Patients who cannot afford expensive hospital and surgical insurance are deprived of the knowledge that there are methods of treatment available for which they can afford to pay, methods which eliminate expensive hospital bills.

3. People who have abnormal fear or religious scruples which prevent their seeking hospital surgery usually try to live with an infirmity rather than seek treatment because they do not know that nonsurgical treatment methods exist.

4. People whose financial situation or work is such that losing even three or four days of employment would seriously disrupt their life style routine are deprived of treatment. This group might include farmers who cannot leave their animals unattended, as well as the man with five or six children whose life would be thrown into havoc by the loss of one paycheck.

5. Elderly people who would be poor surgical risks are denied the possibility of relief without the trauma of a hospital operation.

Change will come in this area. The Federal Trade Commission is concerned about the restraint of price competition resulting from the American Medical Association's ban on advertising by members, and it has served notice that all professions, including doctors, must comply with antitrust laws which prohibit any kind of price fixing. The commission is asking for a change in the code of ethics of the AMA. The commission is asking the AMA to permit advertising that would give patients "a decisional basis for selecting one doctor as opposed to another." It is a change that is long overdue.

XVI

The Land of the Free?

Growing up in Philadelphia in the 1920s and 1930s, I was taught in school what a wonderful form of government we had in the United States. A democracy gives every individual an equal chance, they said. You can rise as high as your talent and ability will take you. Those who are lazy, incompetent, or unproductive will simply not get ahead. Those who have imagination, industry, and initiative will by their efforts improve their lot and their opportunities for advancement; for them, self-fulfillment will be unlimited.

I genuinely believed this until I reached my twenties, when I felt the truth dawn on me, the truth of the adage, "It is not what you know but whom you know." Even the revelation of the world's injustice, however, did not prepare me for what was to happen later. I hate to seem a cynic—and perhaps a bitter cynic, at that—but the story of the loss of my license is one that the osteopathic profession and the Commonwealth of Pennsylvania should certainly be ashamed of. At no time in the twenty-seven years of my practice have I ever given my patients less than 100 percent of my most dedicated effort, and never has one of my over six thousand patients in any way testified against me.

Why was I treated as a criminal if I was innocent? The facts are as I present them. If you raise your head above the crowd, someone in the Establishment will find a way to make it look as if you were guilty of some heinous offense and treat you worse than many who have been convicted of felonies.

151

Numerous doctors each year are convicted of the felony of Medicaid and Medicare fraud but do not lose their licenses. One such physician, the brother of one of the doctors on the board that suspended my license, is presently a fugitive from justice—but his license has never been suspended.

In 1954 Dr. Sam Sheppard was convicted of murdering his wife. He spent the next fourteen years in jail. In 1968 he was released after the now-famous attorney F. Lee Bailey was able to establish a "reasonable doubt" in the minds of a new jury. After his release, this man, who had done no surgery of any kind for fourteen years, was allowed by the Ohio State Board of Medical Examiners and by the authorities of an Ohio hospital to come back and perform very delicate spinal surgery without first taking a refresher course. The results were disastrous. To my knowledge, at least two patients—one middle-aged man and one middle-aged woman—bled to death following surgery performed by Dr. Sheppard.

The heirs of both people sued Sam Sheppard, but the doctor died before either case came to trial, and the question of whether or not there was malpractice in these cases remains unanswered. But some other questions remain as well. Why did the board and the hospital allow this man to return immediately to the practice of surgery? Ordinary prudence on their part certainly would have prevented these two deaths. Ah, but we forget: hospital doctors function under a set of rules different from ours, and the rights of lowly office practitioners can be more fearlessly tampered with.

Lack of competence is reasonable ground for suspension, it seems to me, but licenses are not taken away for that reason—not after fourteen years away from surgery, nor after two extraordinary surgical deaths. Dr. Sheppard was practicing the week he died in April 1970.

Doctors may be known to have histories of drunkenness, may be convicted of fraud, and may be caught doing illegal abortions or selling amphetamine pills to college basketball players, all without losing their licenses. Doctors do not even lose their licenses in proven cases of malpractice. What do you have to do to lose your license? What is the horrendous crime that surpasses all other acts of evil and incompetence in the eyes of the medical profession? As you will learn in the course of my story, the answer is simple: the worst crime of all is advertising.

I entered the osteopathic profession because I wanted to follow in my father's footsteps. My dad, whom I greatly admired, was a selfless osteopathic physician who practiced in Philadelphia for fifty-three years and believed in the efficacy of osteopathic medicine, which he practiced with dedication until the day he died in 1971. When I finished my internship in 1949, I determined that as a D.O. I was not going to be just another doctor—I was going to give the public something distinctive. After all, if the osteopathic profession is not going to give the public a choice, why have a separate profession? Why have two schools of medicine that are identical?

By that time I had already decided that medical molehills were being made into medical mountains and that much unnecessary surgery and hospitalization could be avoided. Without any referral work from hospital-connected practitioners, I tried to build a specialty practice designed to keep people away from surgery and hospitalization. My field was proctology, *i.e.,* rectal diseases, and the nonsurgical treatment of hernia.

Methods of promoting the nature of a doctor's work were well known in the osteopathic profession and had been used by new hospitals and practitioners for many years. Promotional aids being used by the osteopathic hospital in my town, York, Pennsylvania, have been discussed in the preceding chapter, and figure 26 shows an advertisement, long featured in D.O. magazines, promoting a booklet the D.O. specializing in my work might use to publicize his methods of treatment and thus help him build his practice. So promotional aids inviting the attention of the public afflicted with specific diseases had been capitalized on and used for many, many years. This was especially been true for the specialist in ambulant treatment, which, as a little-known field of practice, would not otherwise be considered or understood by the public.

Thus, when I bought my first little booklets on rectal diseases, hernia, and varicose veins from the Journal Printing Company in Kirksville, Missouri, in 1950, they were sent to me without

AN AID TO THE PROCTOLOGIST

Approved by AOA Ethics Committee

We are offering a high grade Proctology Booklet, "Ambulant Treatment of Rectal Diseases," which includes optional pages on Hernia and Varicose Veins. An approved booklet of this type will help your patients to understand what your work is and what it offers sufferers from rectal diseases, ruptures or varicose veins. Write for sample and prices.

JOURNAL PRINTING CO.

KIRKSVILLE, MISSOURI

Fig. 26. An advertisement published in the *Journal of Osteopathy* in February 1959 making informative booklets on ambulant treatment available to physicians. Fifteen years later I was to lose my license for distributing such literature, even though the practice had been considered ethical since early in the century when the above advertisement began appearing.

question. It was considered ethical to inform people by this means, and advertisements making these booklets available for the use of physicians were carried regularly in the *Journal of Osteopathy*.

As my practice grew, patients came to me from greater and greater distances, I treated them successfully and everybody was happy. The patients sent their friends and my feeling of usefulness increased. But not *everybody* was happy. It seems that my patients were going to their family doctors, who were of course connected with hospitals, saying, "Why are you putting your patients in the hospital when Dr. Boyd fixes them in his clinic?"

In 1956 I began to receive in the mail hostile, harassing, and threatening letters from the Pennsylvania Board of Osteopathic Medical Examiners. They told me that I had better stop letting people know about my work, or they would see to it that my hard-earned license to practice my profession would be taken away from me.

This was the state *osteopathic* board! It has always seemed strange to me that a profession started because its founders felt that orthodox medicine was subjecting the public to overtreatment and too much radical treatment would complain when one of its members embarked in a direction of such a conservative nature that it eliminated hospitalization and avoided radical forms of surgery for many common ailments. Have the leaders of this profession thrown away their birthright? Or have they forgotten what the original tenets of osteopathy were?

I am fond of the assertion attributed to Voltaire: "I disapprove of what you say, but I will defend to the death your right to say it." The men on this board were certainly entitled to disapprove of what I was saying, although their supposed philosophy should have caused them to approve and applaud it, but far from defending my right to say it they were proposing to compel me to be silent, or if I would not be silent, to punish me for continuing to express my ideas.

Economist Milton Friedman points out in *Capitalism and Freedom* that the licensure of occupations is rarely instigated by the public to protect them from dishonesty or poor treatment. On the contrary, he explains, the pressure to license comes invariably from members of the occupation itself. And seventy-five percent of the time, it is this same occupational group that gains exclusive control of licensure, as an "agent of the state"—something that is 100 percent true in the field of medicine. The occupational group, thus empowered to license and otherwise regulate practices in the field of their specialty, may then exert control, not for the good of the public, but for the good of the occupation. So there I was, on the verge of losing my license, not because I was a threat to the public, but because I was a threat to the established practices of the licensing group.

I went to my lawyers, who assured me that, yes, these medical politicians did have this great power and if they wished they certainly could remove me from my patients forever. If ever a man thought he was fighting the whole world by himself, I was that man.

Not being a wealthy individual, and with three small children to raise, I took the only course open to me. I shut-up and treated the patients I had, knowing that thousands of suffering people would go to the hospital and go through painful and sometimes mutilating surgery that often was not even successful, because by law I was not allowed to tell them that they could be treated differently. For five years I was a coward and allowed the hospital doctors to make me ashamed of myself as I saw the pain of men seventy or seventy-five, and even a few deaths that may have occurred because I did not have the courage to publicize my proven methods of treatment.

By 1961 I had had enough, and I had my booklet printed again. I advertised in certain newspapers that a free booklet on this type of work could be obtained by writing to a post office box number. Never at any time did my name appear in the ad.

The board was vicious and prompt in their threats and said I would lose my license soon. Apparently there was some disagreement among the board members, or perhaps they did not want any publicity on this matter, because despite constant harassing and threatening registered letters nothing was done until five years later, in 1966, at which time my lawyer and I had to appear before the board in the state capital, Harrisburg, Pennsylvania.

Can you imagine the board bringing the charges and the board also acting as judge and jury? What kind of justice could I expect? The only charge against me of any validity was that I had invited the attention of people afflicted with specific diseases. I freely admitted this and was proud of it; at no time did I deny it.

The board members, not surprisingly, decided that I was guilty as charged. Although my legal costs were growing larger, I had no choice but to fight on.

My attorneys took the case to the appellate court, which in Pennsylvania is called the commonwealth court. For some strange reason, the case was then dropped, and no one knows why. From 1966 until 1973, the board left me alone, and I was no longer made to feel like criminal. What a glorious feeling, just to be allowed to help people and live my life as if I were really a free man.

Alas, I was living in a fool's paradise. The evil forces of the Establishment were not through with me yet, and I was and still am afraid that they will not be satisfied until they have somehow permanently discredited me. I was assured by a friend Vic—York's leading criminal lawyer—that I would win my case in the United States Supreme Court if things ever went that far, so my mind was set a little at ease.

In 1973 I received another letter from the board, stating that I was to lose my license. Again I had to hire lawyers. Again the charges were brought against me by the board, which was again to serve as judge, prosecutor, and jury. Once more I had to stop treating sick people and travel to Harrisburg. Once again the only charge against me was that I had invited the attention of people afflicted with specific diseases. Once again I freely admitted that I was guilty of this heinous crime. Once again not a single patient of mine could be found by the board to say anything against me. Once again the board found me guilty.

In 1974 my expensive lawyers appealed this decision to the commonwealth court. This time the court, composed of seven judges, listened to my case. One of the judges interrupted my lawyer to ask him, "Do you think you should be allowed to advertise?" My lawyer answered no, an answer not surprising from a man who, like most lawyers and doctors, subsists mostly on business from return clients and patients.

But my practice does not work that way. I am constantly discharging patients as cured—never to be seen again. If they do come back, treatment is usually free. Furthermore, there is no legal insurance in this country with discriminatory fee schedules. Every customer pays his own legal bills, and all lawyers function in the marketplace as equals. Not so in my case. My competition is subsidized. A patient with a hernia or with hemorrhoids, for example, can go to the hospital, and his insurance will usually pay his bill. But the insurance company's fee schedule committee, made up of hospital doctors (my competitors), often decides my modest fees are not reasonable, and thus the patient ends up paying a large part

157

of my bill himself. This costs me patients. So I ask, should I not be allowed to advertise, in an effort to make up for such blatant discrimination? Besides, the plain fact is that the public just does not know of the existence of my methods of treatment. My "advertising" aims to make them aware that ambulant treatments exist, that they do have a choice. The Commonwealth Court of Pennsylvania decided unanimously against me.

My lawyers then decided to appeal to the Pennsylvania Supreme Court. Lo and behold, this high and august body of men on large salaries which they will receive in full for the rest of their lives, even after retirement, refused to hear my case. That is, I was guilty.The lower court ruling stood. As a taxpayer and an educated citizen, I resent this. Perhaps I did not expect a fair decision, but I did expect them to hear my case. What are they doing to earn their salaries? By their inaction they participated in taking away a physician's license and did not even care to hear the facts.

The same court ruled one month later that it was legal in Pennsylvania to show *Deep Throat* and other pornographic movies in neighborhood theaters. But it was illegal for a surgeon to tell the public that hospitalization was not required for certain physical ailments.

My lawyers then, for more money of course, decided to take my case to the U.S. District Court in Harrisburg. I had twenty-four patients present in the courtroom to testify for me. I also had the past president of the Pennsylvania Osteopathic Association and two other doctors present to speak in my behalf. The judge stood up in his black robe and looked down upon us, and this great and godly creature said to us poor mortals, "We don't care whether this doctor is a good doctor or a bad doctor. He is guilty of advertising, and we are not going to stand for it."

None of my patients, many of whom had been treated in the hospital unsuccessfully before they consulted me, were allowed to say a thing. My three doctor witnesses were also told that they would not be allowed to testify.

So the next stop, and the next set of expenses, was to take my case to the United States Supreme Court in Washington, D.C. This high and mighty body also decided not to hear my case. The court of last resort turned a deaf ear to a citizen seeking justice. Yet about a month later, this body decided that it was ethical and legal for doctors who did abortions to advertise that fact. Thus we have a decision from our highest court saying that it is legal for doctors to advertise that they do abortions, a procedure that was itself illegal until four or five years ago and may yet become illegal again. But they refused to allow me to keep my license.

So it was that on December 14, 1974, my license was suspended for six months. While I was eating lunch at home the following Monday, four men appeared, two of them in uniform with guns in their holsters. I was told to stop eating and drive with them to my clinic, a request I of course complied with. Inside my clinic they made me take my license off the wall and give it to them, then made me open my wallet, my funds having been depleted by $9,000 in legal fees, and hand over to them the registration card which identified me as a physician. As they were leaving, I showed these minions of the law what a horrible crime I was guilty of, and gave each of them a copy of my clinic booklet.

Headlines two inches high announced the story on the front pages of newspapers in York, Lancaster, and Harrisburg. And the implication was, of course, that the doctor must have been guilty of some type of crime. As usual, the newspapers did not really dig into the story and present the facts. "Doctor Loses License" is sensational; what it does to my reputation does not matter. The newspapers did ask the authorities what would happen to Dr. Boyd if he treated any patients during this six-month period and they were told that Dr. Boyd would be put in jail for ninety days.

I am back in practice now, but many people are afraid to come to me, and my practice has suffered greatly. After all, who wants to go to a doctor who once had his license suspended?

Bibliography

Blanchard, Charles Elton. *A Textbook of Ambulant Proctology.* Youngstown, Oh.: Medical Success Press, 1928.

Blond, Kasper. *Hemorrhoids and Their Treatment.* Baltimore: Williams & Wilkins Co., 1940.

Buie, L. A. *Practical Proctology.* Philadelphia: W. B. Saunders Co., 1937.

Gabriel, William B. *Rectal Surgery.* Springfield, Ill.: Charles C. Thomas, Publisher, 1948.

Goldbacher, Lawrence. *Injection Treatment of Hernia and Hydrocele.* Philadelphia: L. Aubrook & Co., 1938.

Gorsch, R. V. *Perineopelvic Anatomy.* New York: Tilgman Co., 1941.

Hackett, George Stuart. *Joint Ligament Relaxation Treated by Fibro-osseous Proliferation.* Springfield, Ill.: Charles C. Thomas, Publisher, 1956.

Harkins, Henry, and Nyhus, Lloyd. *Hernia.* Philadelphia: J. B. Lippincott Co., 1964.

Harris, F.I., and White, A. S. "Injection Treatments of Hernia." *American Journal of Surgery,* 1937.

Heaton, George. *The Cure of Rupture.* Boston: Houghton, 1877.

Hirschman, L. J. *Handbook of Diseases of the Rectum.* St. Louis: C. V. Mosby & Co., 1936.

Kerr, James, and McPheeters, H. O. *Injection Treatment of Hemorrhoids and Varicose Veins.* Philadelphia: F. A. Davis Co., 1939.

Leden, Hans von; Rand, Robert; and Rinfret, Arthur. *Cryosurgery.* Springfield, Ill.: Charles C. Thomas, Publisher, 1968.

Lovelace, W. R., and Emmett, J. L. "Interprostatic Injections of Sclerosing Solutions." Proceedings of the Staff Meetings of the Mayo Clinic, March 1938.

Rice, Carl O., and Matson, H. "Histologic Changes in the Tissues of Man Following the Injection of Irritating Solutions for the Cure of Hernia." *Illinois Medical Journal,* September 1936.

Riddle, Penn. *Injection Treatment.* Philadelphia: W. B. Saunders Co., 1940.

Shuman, David, with Staab, George. *Your Aching Back and What to Do about It.* New York: Crown Publishers, 1960.

Stanton, Frank D. *Newer Concepts in Clinical Proctology.* Clinton, Mass.: Colonial Press, 1958.

Still, Andrew Taylor. *Osteopathic Research and Practice.* Kirksville, Mo.: Journal Printing Co., 1910.

Still, Andrew Taylor. *Philosophy of Osteopathy.* Kirksville, Mo.: Journal Printing Co., 1899.

Verovitz, C. H. *Diseases of the Veins and Lymphatics of the Lower Extremity.* Boston: Christopher Publishing House, 1941.

Watson, Leigh F. *Hernia.* St. Louis: C. V. Mosby Co., 1948.

Yeomans, Frank C. *Sclerosing Therapy: The Injection Treatment of Hernia, Hydrocele, Varicose Veins, and Hemorrhoids.* Baltimore: Williams & Wilkins Co., 1939.